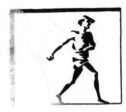

COMPETITIVE FITNESS

Featuring the Officially Licensed Fitness Program of the XIV Olympic Winter Games

By Blair Walliser

SIMON AND SCHUSTER

New York

Published by Simon and Schuster
A Division of Simon & Schuster, Inc.
Simon and Schuster Building
Rockefeller Center
1230 Avenue of the Americas
New York, New York 10020
SIMON AND SCHUSTER and colophon are registered
trademarks of Simon & Schuster, Inc.
Designed by Allan Mogel
Manufactured in the United States of America

10 9 8 7 6 5 4 3 2 1

Library of Congress Cataloging in Publication Data
Walliser, Blair.
    Competitive fitness.

    Includes index.
    1. Physical Fitness.   2. Physical education and train-
ing.   I. Winter Olympic Games (14th: Sarajevo, Bosnia
and Hercegovina)   II. Title.
GV481.W2   1983   613.7′1   83-20389
ISBN 0-671-49800-2

Photo Credits
All photos by Steve Prezant, with the following
exceptions:
Focus on Sports: 12, 16, 17, 18, 19, 20, 21, 23, 25,
26, 27, 28-29, 31, 32, 33, 34-35, 38, 39, 41, 58, 59,
129, 130, 143, 157, 161, 163, 170.
Courtesy of Nautilus Sports/Medicinal Industries
Division: 36, 37
Illustration on page 24 by Amelia McMahon, courtesy
of Doubleday & Co.

Model Fashions by Norma Kamali

CONTENTS

Acknowledgments

With grateful appreciation to Bob Mathias, Director U.S. Olympic Training Center; Bob Beeten, Associate Director, Sports Medicine, U.S. Olympic Committee; Dr. Richard Stedman, Physician to Olympic Ski and Ice Hockey Team; Dr. Richard Levandowski, University Physician, Princeton University; Jack Blatherwick, Olympic Sports Physiologist; Chris Rup, Certified Olympic Athletic Trainer; Jack Moser, U.S. Olympic Committee Sports Medicine Staff; Bob Moore, U.S. Olympic Committee Sports Medicine Staff; and to Steve Hornor, Denny Helwig, Gary Gardiner, Alex Stepanovich, Gordie Genz, John Anderson, Sue Pringle, Mark Fusco, Beth Anders and the many other Olympic coaches, trainers and athletes who patiently gave taped interviews at the U.S. Olympic Training Center.

Thanks also to Bob Bender and Jane Waldman, who offered wise counsel and sound criticism after reading the manuscript, and to Steve Prezant, our brillant photographer, and Russell Hennis, Gery Dinomi, Michelle Joyner and Karla Engels, our athlete models; to Maryanne Travaglione, our physical fitness consultant; and to Steve Adler, Bruce Orosz, Denise Shapiro, the people who made all the arrangements.

A special, affectionate dedication goes to "my four girls," my wife Ursula, and our daughters, Lorian, Tristanne and Bretaigne, who endured the long absences of the head of the family.

FOREWORD

America and most of the rest of the western world are on a fitness kick. It all seems to have begun with a report to President Eisenhower deploring the poor physical condition of America's kids. President Kennedy responded to public concern about the fitness of our youth by appointing The President's Council on Physical Fitness and Sports.

Kennedy also gave us 50-mile walks and touch football games on the White House lawn. The president set an active example for the nation. About ten years later, Frank Shorter, an almost unknown American, won the Olympic gold medal in the marathon. Soon everyone was out jogging; a new craze was born. Bicycles became popular again. A new generation of exercise machines was created, and, as never before, we became body-building conscious.

With this resurgence of general sports interest, a dedicated and determined group of highly competitive young athletes, both male and female, has developed. These young people, eager to compete in the whole range of events, sports, and games, look to this nation's experienced trainers, coaches, athletes, and sports doctors for guidance on the regimens and training routines vital to competitive fitness. This book is a bridge, connecting youthful enthusiasm with seasoned experience—the experience that meets the highest standards in the training methods of our Olympic teams.

INTRODUCTION

The oldest still-standing Olympic records date back to only 1968. In fact, of the more than fifty track, field, and swimming events and almost forty winter events, the records have been broken in nine out of every ten events since 1968. There are two possible explanations:

1. The human body is evolving so rapidly that we are becoming a super race.

2. Our training and nutrition knowledge has expanded so greatly that we are able to get superior performances from the same old human physique.

We have not evolved into super beings, but we have indeed made vast advances in what we know about the body. The popularization of aerobics, for instance, which has had so vast an influence on athletic and general health training, dates back only to 1968. The use of penicillins and antibiotics in the treatment of serious diseases hardly goes back a half century. Many of the dread afflictions that incapacitated so many people either have been eliminated or can now be treated quickly and effectively.

The continued improvement of both men's and women's performances in track, field, swimming, and winter sports events has been due more to our constantly improving knowledge of the body and how it works than to therapies for our ailments. In other days, athletes were given to understand that a diet heavy in protein—more specifically, red meat—was the essence of muscle building. We no longer believe that, because we have learned that carbohydrates are the fuel of the body, and we know that huge, bulging muscles are not the key to record-breaking performances.

In the first modern Olympic Games of 1896, the pole vault was won by William Hoyt, U.S., who hurtled the bar at 10 feet 9¾ inches. In 1924, a vault of 12 feet 11½ by another American, Lee Barnes, was good enough to win the event. Today, all top vaulters are competing to see how far they can surpass the 19-foot bar. Similarly, the time for running the 26.2-mile marathon has been reduced by almost one third since 1896, when a Greek runner was hailed for winning in just under three hours.

Women's Olympic records have fallen similarly. In 1932, the fabulous "Babe" Didrikson won for the U.S. with a javelin throw of 143 feet 4 inches. In recent years, Ruth Fuchs of East Germany has been consistently throwing well over 200 feet, as have her competitors. Time in the 400-meter freestyle relay swim for women has been almost cut in half since 1912.

This all adds up to a simple and unequivocal conclusion: The competitive athlete of today, male or female, in sports or in meet events, must know and observe the most advanced training techniques and must scrupulously follow a well-tailored nutrition plan. The only way for the non-competitive athlete to become competitive in both fitness and performance is to follow the example of the top competitors.

The purpose of this book is to make proven Olympic techniques of body conditioning available to all athletes from their teens on up.

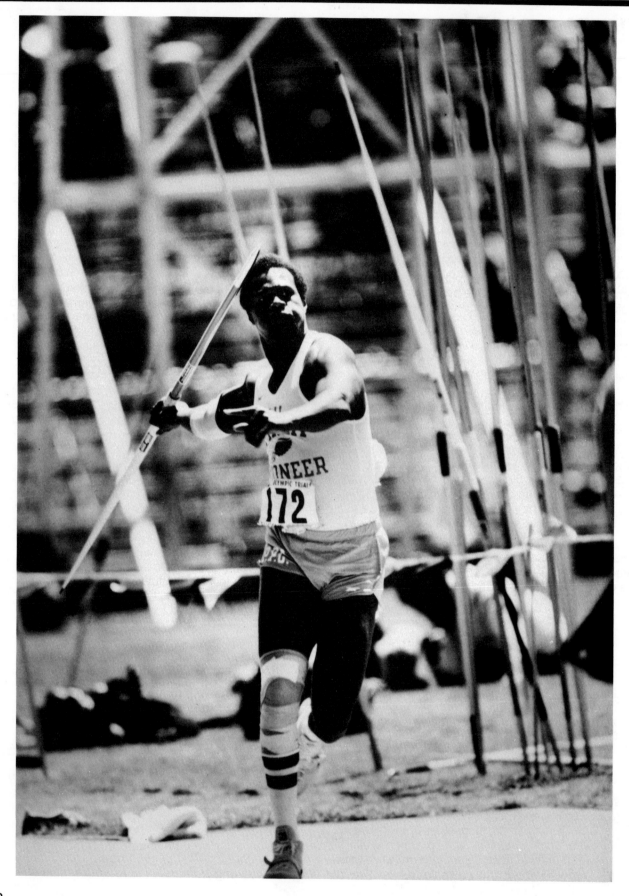

The Olympic Games: A Brief Chronology

9th century B.C. The Greek city states had already established their high regard for physical fitness at the time of Homer, who wrote, "There is no greater glory for a man in his lifetime than that which he wins by his own hands and feet." Footraces, favorites of the Greeks, were run regularly in Elis, on the plain of Olympia. Discus and javelin events were added, and as more cities participated, the event became popular, held every four years.

776 B.C. This year marked both the establishment of the Greek calendar and the establishment of formal record keeping for the quadrennial games at Olympia. The first-known champion was a local boy named Coroebus, said to have been a cook by profession. He won the equivalent of the 200-yard dash (it was officially designated the one-stade race).

480 B.C Xerxes, famed Persian conqueror, landed in Greece with a vast invasion force. When he sent spies to check the Spartan defenders, he was told they were practicing gymnastics, possibly for the Olympic Games. Contemptuous of the Spartans' preoccupation with the games, Xerxes ordered his army to crush them. Three hundred Spartans obliged him by killing some 20,000 Persians before being defeated at Thermopylae.

364 B.C. Tradition forbade any hostilities among the Greek city states during the four weeks of the Olympic Games. In this year, the Elians, who had been ousted as hosts for the games by the Pisates, swept down on Olympia and captured the games—literally.

336 B.C. Alexander the Great is said to have entered a footrace—and lost. The Romans conquered the Greeks and took over the games. Many new events were added, including wrestling, boxing, and the pentathlon. In an early chariot race, Tiberius, who later became emperor, won the event.

66 Nero, Roman emperor, decided to win a few gold medals. He invented some special events (fiddling contests?), which he won. His huge company of fierce bodyguards assured his winning several other events.

Thereafter, contestants poured in from all over the Roman Empire to make the games an international event. Winners were idolized, being granted a free home, free meals for the rest of their lives, and large financial rewards.

388 The last recorded Olympic victor was Prince Varastades, later king of Armenia, who became the boxing champion.

393 Olympia overrun and captured by Goths; sacred shrine destroyed.

394 Emperor Theodosius I abolished the Olympic Games as a pagan spectacle, unsuited for his Christian empire.

1878 Ruins of the ancient Olympic stadium discovered and excavated by Heinrich Schliemann, noted German archeologist, reviving interest in the ancient games.

1896 First modern Olympics for amateur athletes of the world held in Athens.

1912 Jim Thorpe, the great American Indian football star, baseball star, and all-around athlete, won both the decathlon and the pentathlon in the 1912 games in Stockholm. Seven months later, the Olympic Committee took away his medals on the grounds that he had played minor league baseball for $2 a game. After a period of 70 years, the IOC restored Thorpe's medals in 1982 and had his name reinscribed in the record books.

1936 Jesse Owens of the U. S. was one of the earliest of the great black competitors. In 1936, when the Olympics were held in Berlin with Hitler arrogantly proclaiming Aryan supremacy and denigrating all other ethnic types as members of 'inferior races," Owens won four gold medals in the 100- and 200-meter events, the long jump, and the relay. Owens also won world esteem for conducting himself with pride and dignity—much to Hitler's chagrin.

1948 Bob Mathias, athletic director of the 1984 Olympics, won the decathlon in 1948 in London and in 1952 at Helsinki. At 21, he was the youngest ever to win the event.

1956 Al Oerter, U.S. discus thrower, was the only

The five rings of the Olympic symbol stand for the five continents of the world linked by a common desire to excel in athletic competition, governed by the highest ideals of fair play.

The Olympic motto is Citius—Altius—Fortius, which translates from the Latin to mean "Swifter—Higher—Stronger."

athlete ever to win four consecutive gold medals. He captured the discus event in 1956 at Melbourne, in 1960 at Rome, in 1964 at Tokyo, and in 1968 in Mexico City, exceeding his previous mark each time.

1972 Mark Spitz of the U.S. set an all-time Olympic record in 1972 by winning seven gold medals in swimming, three of them in relay events.

Teofilo Stevenson of Cuba was the first contestant to win the heavyweight boxing gold medal three times in a row: 1972, 1976, and 1980.

Held in Munich, the 1972 games were the scene of tragedy when nine Israeli athletes were kidnapped and subsequently killed by Arab terrorists.

1976 Nadia Comaneci of Rumania won the gymnastic competition in 1976 in Montreal with seven perfect scores and endeared herself to millions of television viewers with her wonderful grace.

1980 (winter games) Eric Heiden of the U.S., a speed skater, was the first contestant ever to win five gold medals for individual events. In February of 1980, he scored a grand slam in the men's speed skating events, setting a new record at every distance.

Jim Craig of the U.S. ice hockey team was hailed as a national hero in 1980 when his underdog team took the Olympic title with 6-1-0 record. Craig allowed only 15 goals to opponents in seven games.

1980 (summer games) Alexander Dityatin of the Soviet Union set a slightly tarnished record in the partially boycotted 1980 Games in Moscow by winning eight medals in gymnastics.

These are some of the more important requirements for becoming an Olympic contestant:

1. Good coaching
2. Good facilities: train at a gym or other athletic facility that gives you full opportunity for good workouts
3. Have strong competition as you progress
4. Maintain a healthy mental state: stick with it
5. Practice long, hard hours
6. Be willing to give up a lot of social activity, go to bed early, and stick to a healthy diet when you're in training.
And remember—it's all hard work, no matter what the sport.

—Bob Mathias, director, U.S. Olympic Training Center, and twice Olympic decathlon champion

CHAPTER I: BLOOD, SWEAT, AND FEARS

Nobody remembers the beautifully trained little girl who was runner-up to the charming Nadia Comaneci in the 1976 Olympic gymnastic competition, or the superb swimmer who finished just behind Mark Spitz in the 100-meter freestyle at the 1972 Olympics, or the finely conditioned skater who placed second to Eric Heiden in his record-shattering performance in the 5,000-meter race in 1980. Only one athlete wins in each event, and every contestant offers his or her last ounce of effort and will to be that winner. Also-rans are little noted nor long remembered.

Even so, there is a lifetime of satisfaction in having gained a prized silver or bronze medal and, indeed, in simply having been good enough to take part in the Olympic Games—or any other sports or events that pit you against top competitors and challenge you to excel in fitness, skill, and ability.

There is an even longer-lasting satisfaction for those who maintain their fitness once the days of active competition are over. Part of that satisfaction is good health. The death rate from heart disease is almost twice as high as that from cancer, but cardiovascular exercise is reducing the heart-attack rate. Keeping fit may mean living longer.

The first essential element of athletic fitness—and fitness for the rest of your life—is cardiovascular conditioning (and co-relative with that, respiratory conditioning). These are the two requisites for endurance and stamina, which are in turn prime requisites for success in both Olympic events and popular sports.

The kind of maximum effort that wins track and field events requires the delivery of large amounts of oxygen to the muscle systems of the body to help fuel them for their top performance. The oxygen is delivered by the blood, which in turn is pumped by the heart. The stronger the muscles of the heart, the more blood it can pump—provided the blood vessels are large enough to permit the flow. One reasonably healthy heart can pump as little as three quarts of blood a minute; another may pump up to twelve quarts. If your blood vessels are twice as large as another person's, they will transport four times as much blood.

Cardiovascular conditioning strengthens the heart muscles and increases the capacity of the blood vessels. Even at rest, the well-conditioned heart is superior in performance, generally beating at least ten times a minute less often than the flabby heart. This can amount to 5,000 fewer beats in the course of a good night's sleep. The well-conditioned heart will use less effort in delivering blood and oxygen to the muscles and tissues to help refuel them as they burn up energy.

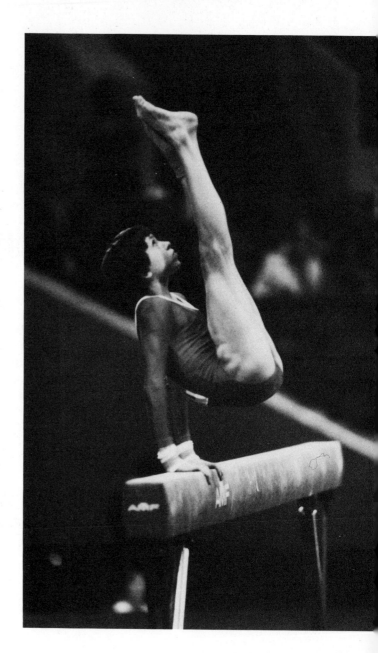

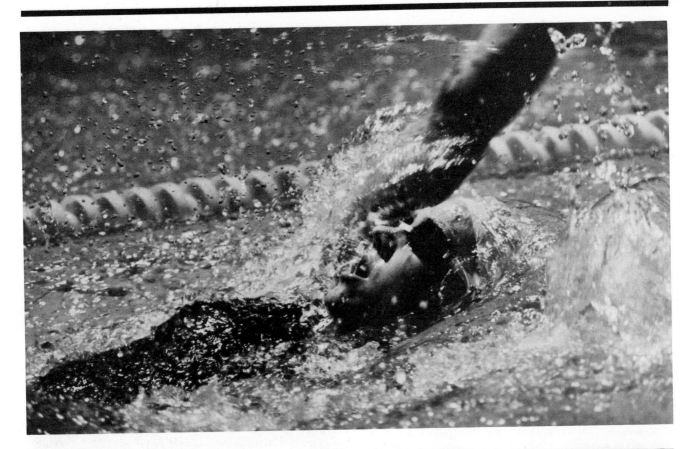

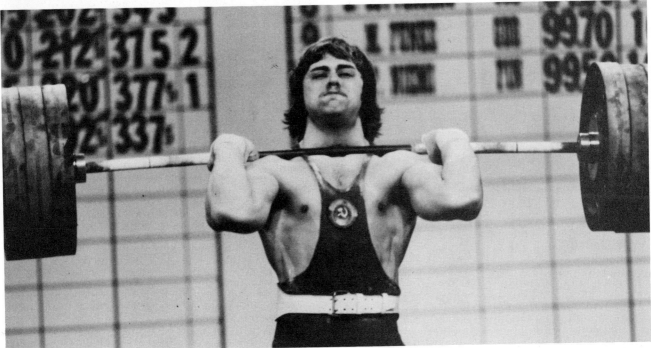

I think one of the reasons we continue breaking records is that our nutrition and diet knowledge is so much improved. So we have a better base to start from.
—Bob Beeten, associate director, sports medicine, U.S. Olympic Training Center

The fitness of your circulatory system is important not only in athletics but in almost all daily activities. If your brain doesn't get enough blood, you may blackout or suffer memory loss. If your kidneys or liver don't receive enough blood, they malfunction. If you're losing your hair, it may be due to poor circulation to the scalp. And if you're eager for an active love life, you'd better be certain that the circulation that supplies blood to your sex organs is functioning efficiently. In a phrase, take care of your heart if you expect it to take good care of you.

Closely related to cardiovascular conditioning is respiratory conditioning. The body cannot store oxygen. As muscular effort increases, more and more oxygen is consumed. This oxygen is derived solely from the amount of air taken in and processed by the lungs. An athlete in top condition may be able to process air twice as fast as someone in poor condition. The athlete's well-conditioned heart will show a pulse rate of ten to twenty beats slower per minute than a poorly conditioned competitor. It is this reserve power of heart and lungs in time of intense effort that separates winners from also-rans.

Along with conditioning of the heart and lungs must go conditioning of the muscles. Conditioning converts flabby, ineffective muscle tissue to firm and powerful tissue. Fat is replaced by sinew. Muscles increase in size and capability only by being regularly pushed to the limits of their ability; they can only advance beyond their present limits by being constantly pushed to superior performance, which means pushing the heart and lungs to similar extreme limits.

This pushing to the outer limits involves a risk. You must have passed a thorough physical examination before you get involved in rigorous conditioning, and you must have regular examinations at least once a year to be certain that you are physically up to the strains that intensive conditioning places on the body.

We have now noted the first three elements of athletic fitness: the heart, the lungs, and the muscles. There is a fourth element that also demands intense application—training in agility and flexibility. Flexibility means that muscles and tendons remain limber in their range of motion about a body joint. Flexibility is attained by stretching all of the various muscle groups of the body in turn. Stretching

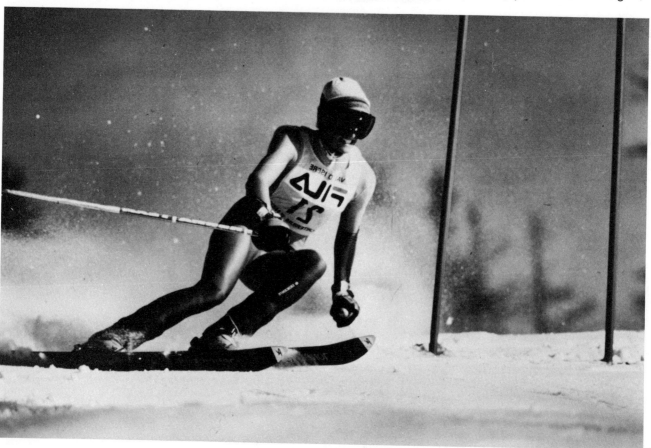

The only pressure I feel is knowing I'm going to punish my body terribly out there.
—*Eric Heiden,* The Olympian, *March 1979*

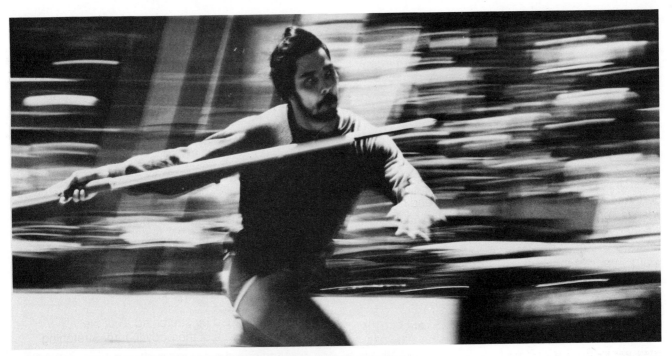

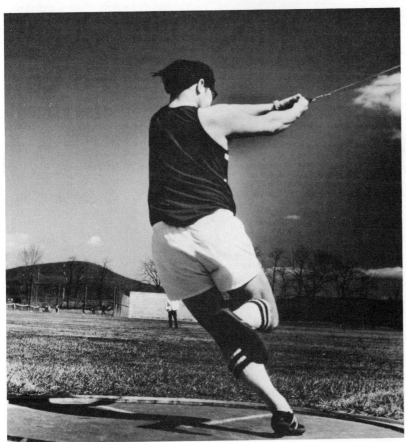

must be done regularly and systematically.

Agility implies rapidity, dexterity, and lightness. Is it possible for a big man to be "light" and "agile?" Watch a defensive back break through for a quarterback sack or a 7-foot 2-inch center pull a rebound off the backboard, and you'll realize that size is no barrier to agility. Speed, balance, coordination, and fast reflexes all go into agility. They must all be cultivated in a training regimen that pushes the body always toward faster and more intense responses to stimuli.

We will take up the subject of the psychological factor in competition later, but mental conditioning is an important element in developing fast reflexes and muscular coordination. From our prehistoric ancestors we have inherited the reaction to danger that is commonly called "fight or flight." First comes the alarm signal and instantaneously, the adrenal gland starts pumping the hormonal secretion adrenaline into the blood stream. Blood pressure bounces up, the heart action spurts blood throughout the body as the blood vessels dilate, and both metabolism and muscular contractions sharply increase. Your body is on the alert for immediate action; the adrenaline has mobilized your physical and mental resources for fast action. In such a situation, a 120-pound woman has been known to lift the rear end of a car so that her son could be removed from underneath.

Athletes know the advantages of being "psyched up." But the important thing to remember is that the amount of stimulation should be proportionate to the effort at hand. David was not bursting with energy when he fired his slingshot; he was cool and controlled. A hunter facing a charging bear, with only one shot remaining in his rifle, may be hyped with adrenaline, but he keeps his cool if he wants to keep his life. Athletes generally agree that they perform best when they're nervous and even a little queasy before their event. This anxiety does not represent a risk—it seems to be a necessary prelude to maximum effort. The successful competitor recognizes this state of mind and uses it to draw the maximum speed, coordination, strength, and balance from his body. In his all-out competitive challenge, he mobilizes his fears to support the weeks and months of training that have all pointed toward this test of his abilities.

The road to competitive athletic fitness—and particularly to Olympic levels of fitness—is thus a matter of blood, sweat, and fears. The blood, charged with fresh oxygen, must be delivered to the muscles when demanded, which calls for intensive training of the cardiovascular and respiratory systems. This provides the endurance and stamina. The sweat must be spent to achieve muscular size and power, combined with coordination and agility. And the fear that must be controlled—the fear of failure, of not being quite good enough—must be faced, must be endured, and must in the end be made part of the winning effort.

Our gymnasts and figure skaters continue to get younger and younger. Their parents must serve as a supportive mechanism—but not as a control.

Parents must be careful not to be oversupportive, trying to have vicarious athletic careers and win glory through their children.
—Bob Beeten, associate director, sports medicine, U.S. Olympic Training Center

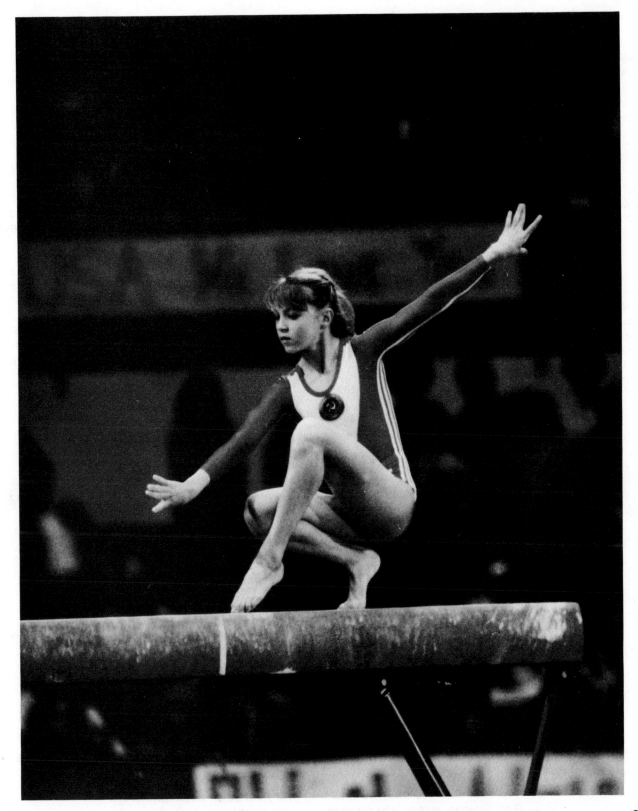

CHAPTER II: THE HUMAN BODY

The human body is the most marvelously complex and ingenious mechanism in the world. If we had to learn to operate our bodies the way we learn to operate a computer, it would take us years of exhausting practice, and we would never become very good at coordinating the infinite activities that nature has programmed us to do without thinking. To name only a few:

Maintaining a regular heartbeat (increasing as needed)
Breathing regularly
Digesting food and eliminating waste
Replacing dead and dying tissue with fresh tissue
Sweating, shivering, tensing, relaxing
Registering and interpreting sense perceptions
Controlling bodily movements
Maintaining the body at a constant temperature
Lubricating mouth and throat; oiling the skin

The highly complex muscular and circulatory systems are based around and supported by the frame—the skeletal system. Without the skeleton, we'd be a race of jellyfish. The skeleton supports the muscles, protects vital organs, permits mobility of the limbs and head, and manufactures blood in the bone marrow. The digestive system converts food to fuel or human energy.

A woman requires less food intake than a man by about 250 calories because she tends to weigh less and to use less energy. A woman of average size uses up about 1,400 calories a day to sustain her basic life processes—breathing, heartbeat, digestion, and circulation. An average man will use up 1,650 calories on these same involuntary functions. A woman or man can burn up 320 calories an hour walking and 600 calories running or jogging.

The average woman is a little under 5 feet 4 inches tall and weighs 135 pounds.

The average man is about 5 feet 9 inches tall and weighs about 172 pounds.

Of course, "average" people are extremely rare, but these figures suggest why men's Olympic records tend to surpass women's records by 12 to 20 percent and why women are not required to compete against men.

Within the limits of gender, nature has engineered some other variables. These are known as somatotypes, or body shapes. The broad general divisions are:

Endomorphs —heavy-set people
Mesomorphs —well-built, muscular people
Ectomorphs —slim, smaller-boned people

There are few people who exactly conform to any of these general body types. Rather, we tend to be somewhere in between, with one or another type predominating. We cannot choose or change our body types, because they originate in our heredity— our genes—but we can modify them slightly by our habits and conditioning. For instance, an ectomorph who grows up as a skinny stringbean can, by developing powerful muscles, assume some of the aspects of the athletic mesomorph. So, too, can the burly endomorph trim himself into a muscular physique. For this, you must start early—in the mid teens.

For fitness training purposes, the muscles of the body can be divided into three major groups:

The Upper Body
Shoulder muscles: Trapezius, Deltoids
Arm, Wrist, and Hands: Biceps and Triceps, Extensors
Chest: Pectoralis, Serratus

The Mid Body
Waist: Abdominals, Intercostals, Obliques
Back: Spinal Erectors, Latissimus Dorsi, Sacrospinalis

The Lower Body
Buttocks: Gluteus Maximus and Minimus, Iliotibial, Fascio Gracilis, Abductor Magnus
Thighs: Quadriceps and Biceps Femoris, Adductors, Sartoris, Hamstrings
Calves: Gastrocnemius, Extensors, Tibialis Anterior
Ankles and Feet: Achilles Tendon, Plantar

Olympic athletes have learned to take harder and harder stress and strain. But there is always a point of diminishing returns—and each athlete has to learn where that point is by what his body tells him. The average elite competitor trains five to seven days a week for the Olympics with double-day (twice a day) workouts and sometimes even triple-day workouts. A good deal of that is not intensive but at the skill level.

—Bob Beeten, associate director, sports medicine, U.S. Olympic Training Center

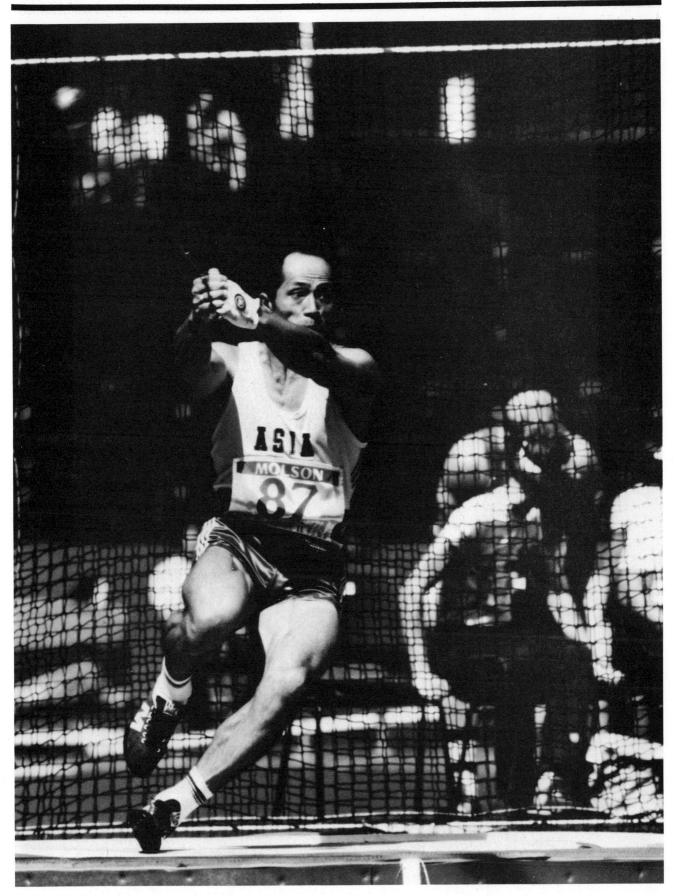

SKELETAL MUSCLES (Frontal View)

SKELETAL MUSCLES (Dorsal View)

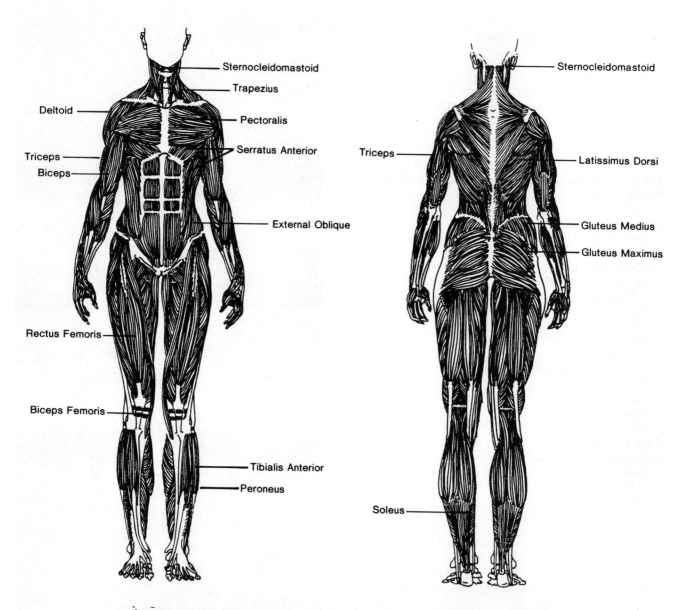

Sternocleidomastoid

Trapezius

Deltoid

Pectoralis

Serratus Anterior

Triceps

Biceps

External Oblique

Rectus Femoris

Biceps Femoris

Tibialis Anterior

Peroneus

Sternocleidomastoid

Triceps

Latissimus Dorsi

Gluteus Medius

Gluteus Maximus

Soleus

I was an artistic gymnast for three years and I was pretty strong. But I think I had a mental block. I was scared, maybe because I was so young. I took rhythmic gym to improve my flexibility, dance, and grace. I found it was more "me"—I'm really more of a dancer than a tumbler.

The Europeans have had this sport for ages, and it's only been here in the U.S. for eight or ten years. But we're doing pretty well—I think we'll show them!

—Michelle Berube (17), national champion, rhythmic gymnastics

Of the three essential elements of the body—bone, muscle, and fat—the bones are least subject to conditioning. The vertebral column, the femur and tibia, the pelvis cannot be lengthened or thickened. A careful diet, adequate in mineral and vitamin content, is the best treatment for the bones. However, careful conditioning of the muscles can maintain the skeleton in its most efficient form and help to avoid functional disorders like stiffness or arthritis of the joints, the round shoulders brought on by poor posture, and the so-called hollow chest, attributable to prolonged sitting and the languid slump common to office workers. Over a long period, functional displacement like the slump or the round-shoulder effect can eventually become structural.

All of the muscle groups of the body can be divided into three types. The body muscles mentioned above are known as voluntary muscles because they are controlled by an act of will. These muscles can all be developed and conditioned by the training exercises that will be described in following chapters.

There are also involuntary muscles, which are not subject to conscious control. Sometimes called smooth muscles, they line the digestive tract and power the blood vessels. They do their job automatically, whether you're awake or asleep.

The third type of muscle, also involuntary in its action but responsive to the mind and will at times of great stress, is the cardiac muscle, the muscle that makes the heart beat. The involuntary muscles are subject to development only through aerobic exercise, such as running. A whole range of anaerobic exercises—weight training, for example—calculated to build power in the skeletal muscles will have almost no effect on the involuntary muscles. The training regimen of the competitive athlete must include both types of exercise.

The final component of the body, in addition to muscle and bone, is fat. An "ideal" weight table, as developed by American insurance companies, can be checked for reference. However, many heavily muscled athletes might be considered overweight based on these statistics. The real check is the pinch test. Pinch any part of your mid body between the thumb and forefinger: If you find more than an inch easily pinchable, the likelihood is that some of that is fat. With the possible exception of the long-distance (English Channel-type) swimmer, the body does not need stored-up fat for competitive athletic events. Stay on a weight-control diet and use up the fat in strenuous training exercises. (Some trainers maintain there is no way to lose fat permanently except through a continuing exercise regimen.)

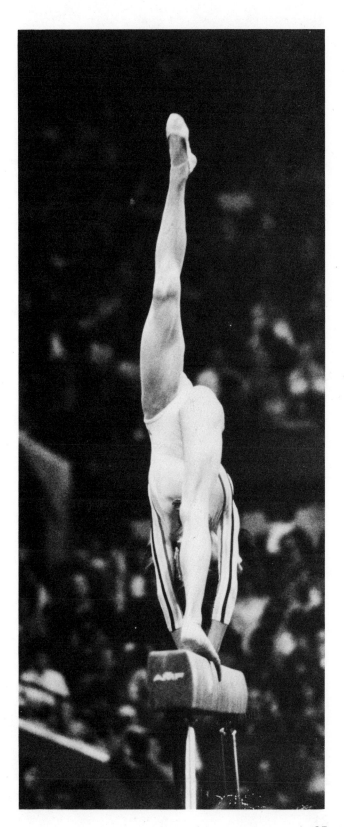

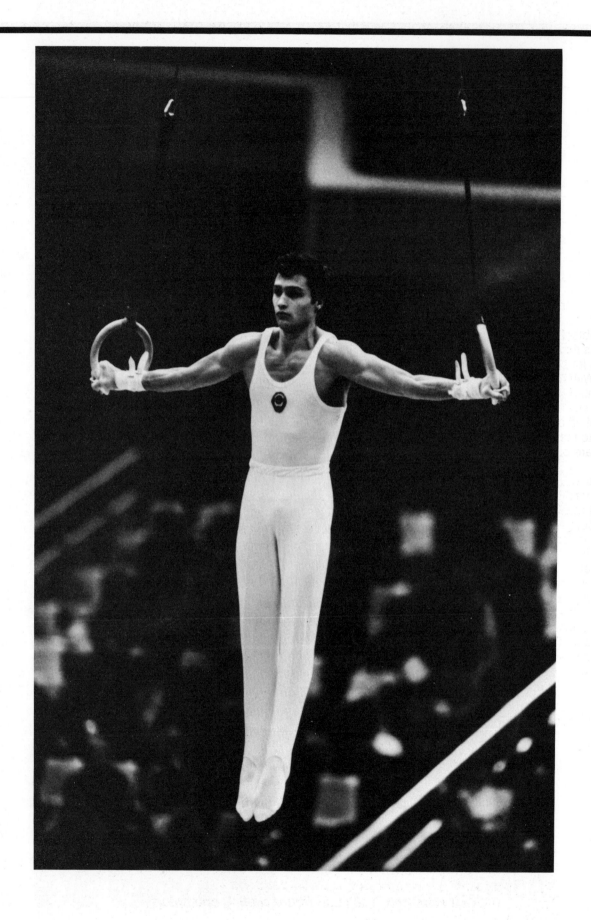

There is a further component of competitive fitness, one which is inherent in the body but is not physical—the psychological factor. In a phrase, it's "getting it all together" to make the supreme effort—and the effort is directed at winning, only at winning. From what we know of the ancient Olympic Games, there were no awards for second or third place.

Winning is what it's all about, claim many coaches, citing the much-quoted aphorism attributed to the late great football coach Vince Lombardi: "Winning isn't everything—it's the only thing." Those who knew Lombardi as an advocate of fair play and good sportsmanship on the field do not interpret this as an injunction to the athlete to win by any means possible, fair or foul. What Lombardi was saying, they feel, is that you never train for, expect to achieve, or strive for anything less than victory.

With rare exceptions, there is almost never an undefeated champion in sports. Even the strongest runners, skiers, divers, and weight lifters have occasional off days. The consistent winners are those who go into the game or event with the conviction that they are capable of winning. Are they nervous before they start? Almost universally. But they do not let the stress and anxiety reach a peak where it pours adrenaline into their veins long before it's needed or allows tense muscles to vitiate the fine edge of fitness. The old routine of doing push-ups, sprints, and deep kneebends to allay tension may relax the mind, but it also tires the muscles. Some athletes hone their concentration by a meditation technique with which they shut out their surroundings and visualize a soft blue rectangle with a single white cloud floating across it. Other athletes mentally rehearse the start, the game plan, and the victorious finish. These methods may not scare the butterflies away, but at least they help the contestant to keep from dwelling on all the things that could go wrong.

In every contest, there is only one winner; some defeats are inevitable. The true psychological edge is achieved by the athlete who studies the event, learns what he did wrong and what he did right, and uses the experience to improve his showing the next time out.

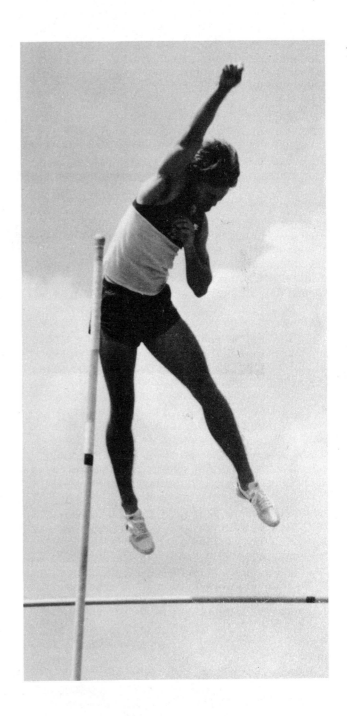

You can't miss a practice. You don't want to. You want everybody to think you're a machine. And sometimes you are—hopefully, at competitions. A machine is geared to do a particular job and is very efficient at it. If you have a good week of practice before a competition, you have a good competition.
—*Scott Hamilton, 1983 U.S. figure skating champion*

CHAPTER III: TRAINING FOR TRAINING

No one ever talks about going into training for going into training, but it's an extremely important subject. At the heart of a good conditioning program is a regular schedule. Not an ideal schedule—a "super" schedule or a "farthest limit" schedule—but a practical schedule that, with a little strain, you can follow regularly and accurately. If you're already into an organized conditioning regimen with guidance from an experienced coach or trainer, you might find it useful to compare this chapter for possible improvement of your present effort. If not—then let's train our sights on training for training.

First of all, you must set a regular time. If you have a workout schedule at a gym, that time is already set. If not, select a time of day and days of the week when you are least likely to be interrupted, disturbed, or distracted. Some athletes like to get out early in the morning, especially in summer. You'll see them jogging, skipping rope, and stretching in the parks, along rivers, on country roads—and, yes, on city asphalt—practically from dawn on. Others make time at lunch hour or after work. And still others find late evening, just before going to bed, a good private time. The absolute no-no is too soon after a meal.

If you find that your daily schedule doesn't easily fall into a pattern, you may be better off joining a group or working out at an established fitness center. Most of us are strongly influenced by group pressures. If the weather's bad or we're feeling pooped, the knowledge that others are expecting us to join in with them exerts a strong moral suasion on our faltering will. Remember that the schedule you set up is not for this week or this month, but for this year—and possibly, in one form or another, for many years to come. You may want to do your aerobic conditioning—jogging, rope skipping—outside. Swimming, of course, requires access to a pool. But your calisthenics and weight work requiring particular equipment must be done in a gym or in a room at home large enough to permit freedom of motion.

To many people, having an attractive outfit for working out furnishes a strong added incentive. So be it. This may be one of the few contributions that fashion designers have made to the national welfare. In a recent survey, a popular women's magazine discovered that 42 percent of the magazine's readers engaged in body conditioning from time to time; 51 percent had bought some kind of exercise equipment; and over 80 percent had bought special clothing!

The most important thing about the special clothing is not the color, design, or dashing stripes and patterns but that the outfit be loose and comfortable enough to allow perfect freedom of movement and

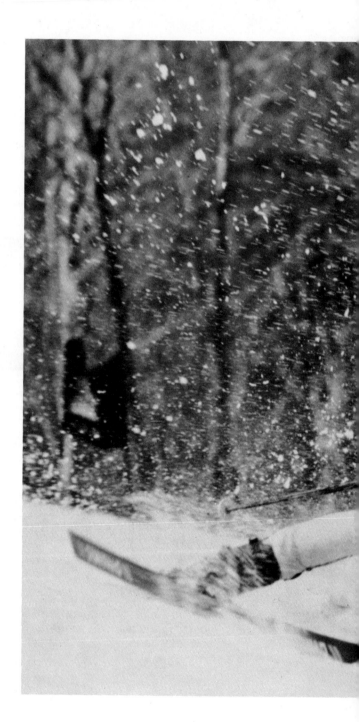

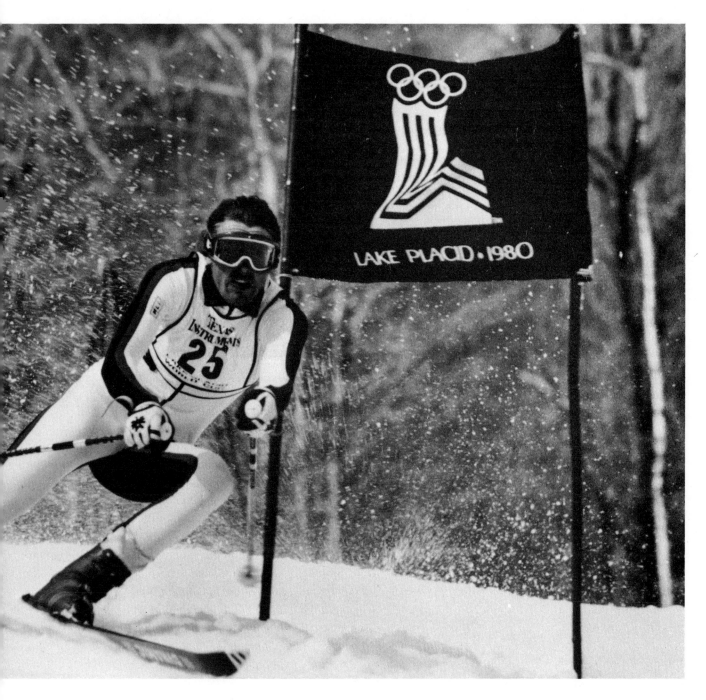

Weight lifting and strengthening used to be for a select few. A lot of sports people thought you lost agility through weight lifting, but that's been proven false. With proper weight-lifting techniques, you can use weight lifting to gain weight or to lose weight, to gain strength and to gain flexibility. It is one training routine I would recommend to any young athlete.
—Steve Hornor, soccer trainer

that it absorb perspiration while permitting air circulation through to the skin. The same applies to bras and athletic supporters.

If any part of your workout clothing is to be accorded money and thought, it's your shoes. They should fit perfectly, should support the instep, and yet should give freely with the motion of the foot. Most athletes wear two pairs of socks—a close-fitting, absorbent inner pair and a heavier outer pair. This provides maximum protection against chafing and blistering. Whenever any part of your foot shows signs of chafing, it's a good idea to change your shoes or sock combination at once. A good foot powder applied before workout is helpful if your feet are especially sensitive. If you have any tendency toward athlete's foot, take special care to wash well with soap between the toes while showering.

Before you start to stock up on equipment for home or backyard workouts, you'll want to canvass the exercises recommended for your sport. You probably won't need a full set of barbells if your specialty is the marathon, and you almost certainly will need an exercise bicycle if you have no place to run outdoors.

A good item to start with is an exercise mat, since many fundamental exercises require applying various parts of the anatomy to the floor. The surface you exercise on should not be too hard, rough, or dirty to be comfortable.

A good set of barbells with weight disks capable of graduated combinations is available at most sporting goods stores, as are dumbbells and foot weights. For women, a set of easily grasped, rounded hand weights will be helpful. A good, well-made jump rope should be part of your equipment; the light children's kind is all but useless.

A number of exercises call for a light rod about 4 to 5 feet long. A section of clothes pole or a broomstick will do. Many of the exercises can be done with a chair, a sofa, or a bureau. A pair of sturdy wooden—or plastic—boxes that will readily support your weight is handy to have. If you have room enough to store (and money enough to afford) an exercise bench with a weight rack and other attachments, you'll find it useful. If your funds are unlimited, you can think of a rowing machine and one of the various multi-exercise machines. We'll presume that you already have a record player or tape deck with access to bright, lively music for some of the repetitive workout routines.

Are you ready now to hit the fitness trail with a disciplined routine and a long-term plan for reaching peak performance? Not unless you've had a physical examination by a competent medical authority or

Sometimes I feel I should have a battery pack with me to recharge myself. What's tough is that everyone's always looking for something better from me. But I take it as a challenge. I just try to do the best and most consistent job I can.
—Greg Lougannis, 10-meter platform diving champion

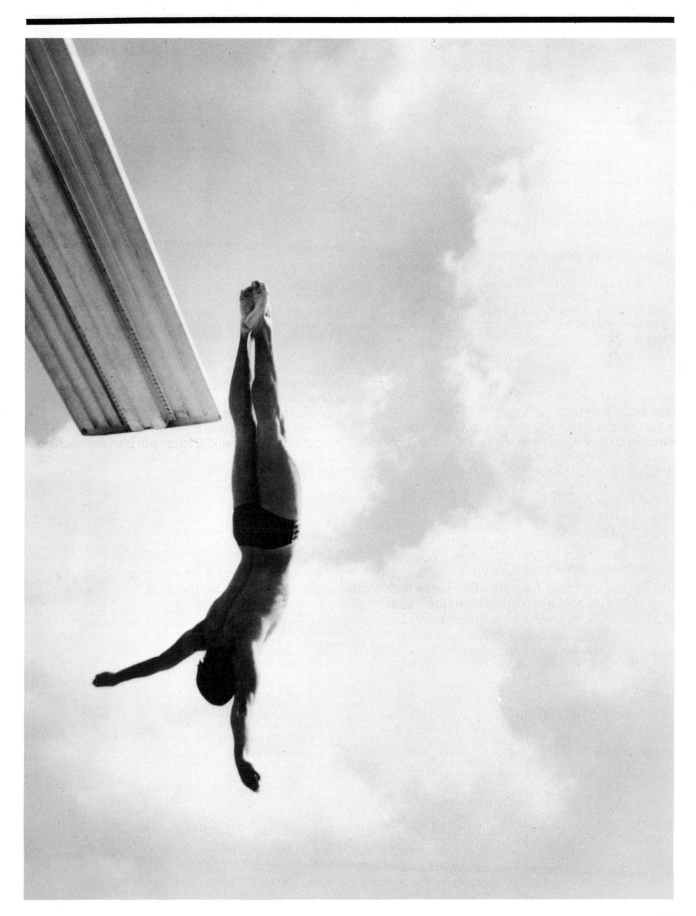

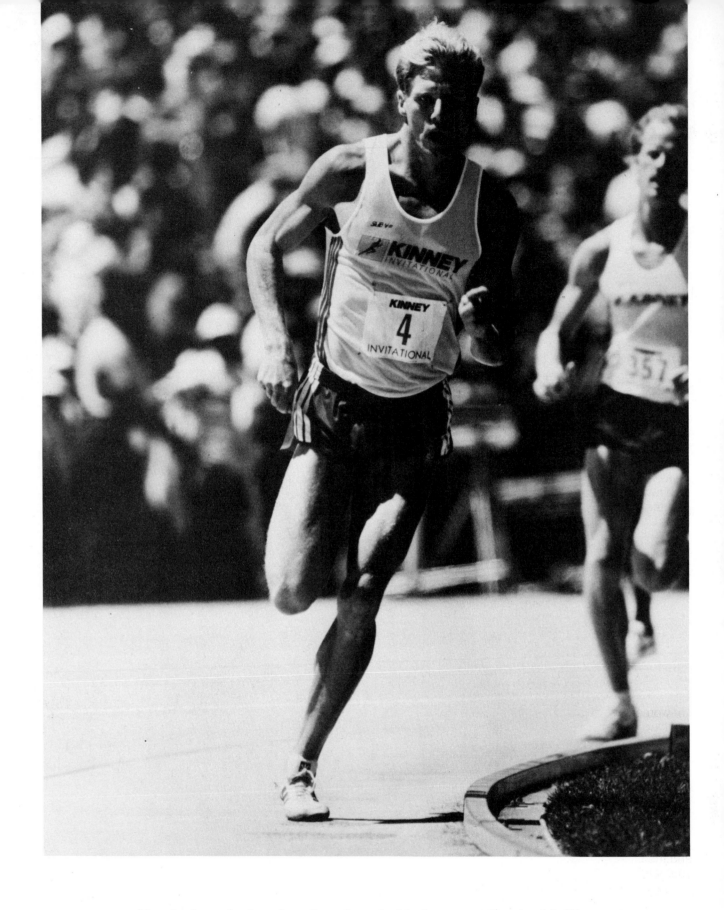

The doctor asked me how long I wanted to keep running. I said, "Forever!"
—Francie Larrieu-Smith, after winning the gold medal in the
1500-meter run at the National Sports Festival with a nerve-shattered,
bandaged foot.

sports doctor within a year's time and have been given a bright-green go-ahead. The upcoming routines are not for the weak hearted, those with a respiratory condition, or victims of some kinds of organic malfunction. Make sure—take the exam.

After that, are you ready? Not quite. It's a good idea to find out just where you stand in your present fitness shape. One of the simplest, most direct tests is the Air Force Aerobics test devised by Maj. Kenneth Cooper. He found it worked on virtually everyone, from teenagers through Air Force personnel up to senior citizens.

The test consists of determining the utmost distance that you can travel on foot in 12 minutes. Here's how Cooper describes it: "We furnish the time: 12 minutes. You furnish the distance. Please keep in mind that it's a maximum test, and that it's your body being tested. I can't run behind you with a pitchfork to keep you going. You've got to push yourself very close to exhaustion. . . . Start out running, but if your breath gets short, walk for a while until it comes back, then run some more. Keep going for the full 12 minutes." You should not even attempt this test if you aren't already in training.

When you've checked the distance (either by running on a measured track at a school or gym or by measuring it on your car speedometer), you can refer to the following table for your rating:

Distance Covered in 12 minutes	Fitness Category
less than 1.0 mile	Very poor
1.0 to 1.24 miles	Poor
1.25 to 1.49 miles	Fair
1.50 to 1.74 miles	Good
1.75 miles or more	Excellent

For women, the good-fitness category is indicated as anything over 1.30 miles in 12 minutes, and for men over 35, it's anything over 1.40 miles.

The Air Force test is essentially a respiratory (aerobic) check. An excellent cardiovascular check is the Tecumseh Step Test, which you may have taken in your doctor's office. It consists of stepping up on to and down from a box 8 inches high at the rate of 24 steps a minute for 3 minutes. After you've finished the three minutes (72 on-off steps), you wait exactly one minute and then take your pulse. The following table gives your rating:

Man's Pulse	Woman's Pulse	Rating
68 or under	76 or under	Excellent
68–79	76–85	Good
80–89	86–94	About Average
90–99	95–109	Below Average
100 or over	110 or over	Very Poor

The maximum human heart rate is accepted as 220 beats per minute. The maximum for any given individual is accepted as 220 beats per minute minus his or her age. The main principle of aerobic training is to build your pulse rate up to 70 percent of your maximum and then hold it there. The aerobic benefits begin about 5 minutes after the exercise starts, and they continue for as long as you exercise. The Air Force prefers a minimum heartbeat of 150 per minute for active athletes while exercising. Only the most strenuous exercises will produce this rate; these are called aerobic exercises. They are exercises that use up a lot of oxygen (the word *aerobic* comes from a Greek word for "air"). Aerobics are the kind of strenuous exercises, such as biking, swimming, or running, that enable your lungs to produce enough oxygen to fuel your body and your heart and blood vessels to become strong enough to deliver the increased amounts of blood to provide the oxygen for maximum effort. There are five other types of exercises which may require skill, muscular power, and endurance but are generally anaerobic in that they do not directly develop the cardiovascular and respiratory systems.

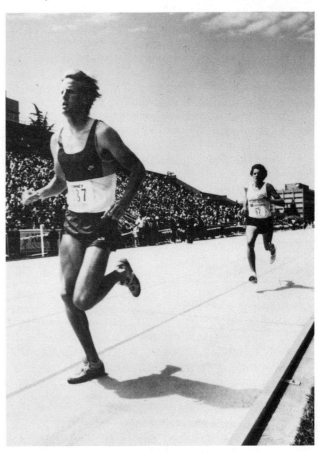

Calisthenics

Calisthenics are what most people refer to when they talk about "doing exercises." The word comes from two Greek words meaning "beauty" and "strength." The concept of achieving beauty and symmetry of body through fitness training has a long and honorable history. Calisthenics is a rather broad and vague term that includes "setting-ups" but may also include three more precise forms of exercise, isometrics, isotonics, and isokinetics.

Isometrics

Shortly after World War I, a group of scientists working to analyze muscle function tied down one leg of a frog to determine how long it would take for the leg to atrophy from lack of exercise. What was their astonishment to find that after several weeks the tied leg was actually stronger than the free one! From this they drew the now accepted conclusion that a muscle straining against an immovable object—including an opposing muscle of the same body—could be developed in size and strength without motion. An exercise is said to be *isometric* when it involves effort expended against an immovable object.

When you press your hands together as hard as you can and tense one arm against the other until you literally quiver, this is isometric exercise. Another isometric exercise is to place your hands behind your head and press hands against head and head against hands as hard as you can. Or just sit still in your chair and flex one set of muscles after another, as hard as you can in sequence around the body. Isometrics became a popular fad because they promised fitness in minimum time without stirring from your chair. Today, isometric exercise is accepted as part of training, but it must be done in conjunction with isotonic and isokinetic workouts.

Isotonics

If your goal is muscle building, your answer is isotonics. However, it should be pointed out that sheer muscle size has very little to do with competitive fitness except in the weight-lifting events. In our society, which relies heavily on appearances, muscularity tends to be equated with masculinity and sexual prowess. This theory is not documented by scientific research.

The famed Milo of Crotona, an archetypal Olympic winner, was the first recognized practitioner of isotonics. He lifted the same calf every day for a year after

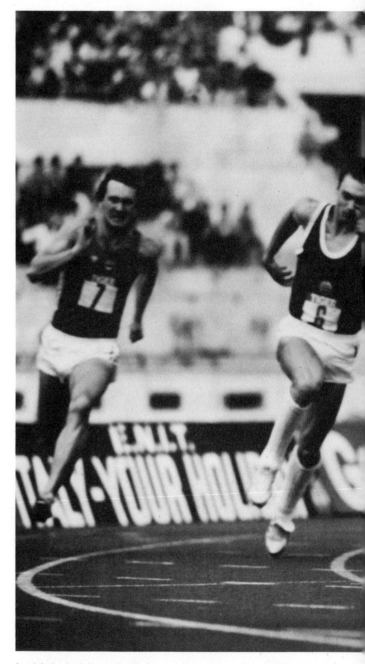

its birth. In his daily hefting of a mass of beef, from day-old calf-hood to year-old bull-hood, he also anticipated weight training. He was acclaimed as the strongest man in the world of his day. His Olympic victories, however, were gained in the beefcake categories, not in sprinting, leaping, or throwing. A classic example of the distinction between isometrics and isotonics may have been the giant Atlas. As long as he groaned and supported the earth on his back, that

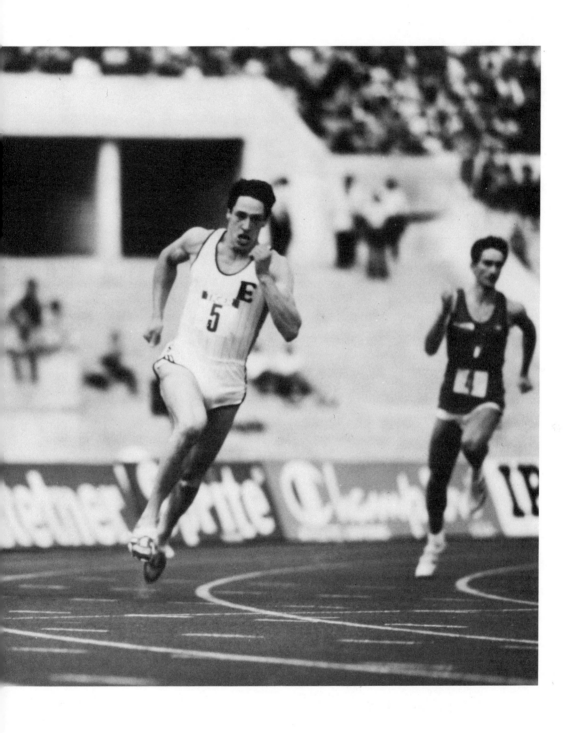

You've got to keep pushing your body harder. When I'm running, I feel like I'm the jockey, and my body is the horse.
—Cliff Wylie, 400-meter contestant

was isometric; when he cleverly tossed it to Hercules, that was isotonic.

This is not to minimize the value of isotonic exercise. Power lifting involves the use of barbells in the bench press, squat, and dead lift. The Olympic lifts are somewhat different and are classified as the Snatch and the Clean and Jerk. Since isotonic exercises fundamentally consist of moving a weight against gravity, the push-up, sit-up, and chin-up may properly be included. The chief drawback in depending too heavily on these exercises is that they do not develop the speed and agility required in most competitive athletics. They form a part of training but are not a fitness regimen in themselves.

Isokinetics

Isokinetic exercise differs from isotonic in that it provides a variable resistance for a muscle or muscle group to work against while permitting a range of movement for the joint about which the muscles may be acting. When you move a weight against gravity, it's easier at certain points and more difficult at others. Variable resistance is provided by a machine that assures equal stress on the muscle throughout the range of its motion.

The two machines that have gained most acceptance for isokinetic exercise are the Nautilus and the Universal. The Nautilus has a range of devices adapted to training for a variety of muscle groups. The big advantage of this kind of training is that it helps you to develop strength at fast speeds, far better suited to the kind of power you need in sports than simple muscle bulge. Nautilus equipment is expensive and is usually found at special training centers developed by Nautilus. "Full range exercise" is their claim.

The Universal Gym is most often found at Ys, high schools, and colleges. It too supplants weight-lifting equipment but does not have the range or versatility of the Nautilus. The counsel and programming of a coach or trainer is recommended when using such machines in training for a special sport or event.

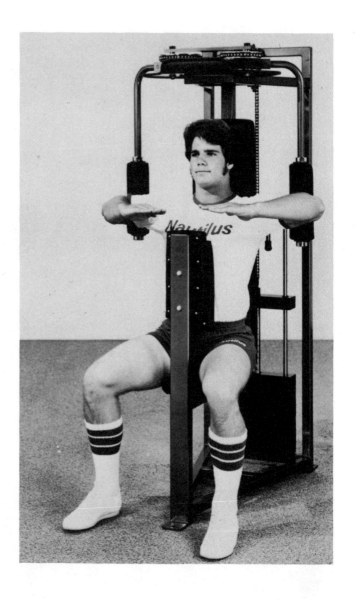

I'm thinking positive thoughts all the time. I never allow anything negative to enter my mind. During training or warm-ups, I certainly don't want anyone suggesting "You can't do it." A lot of weight lifting is mental. People just aren't getting all they can out of their bodies. When I get ready to lift, I'm thinking positive—I'm always thinking, "I'm going to make it!" I perceive the image of making it. And then, of course, the crowd gets you pumped up.
—Curt White, NSF gold medal winner and record holder in the 82.5 kg class

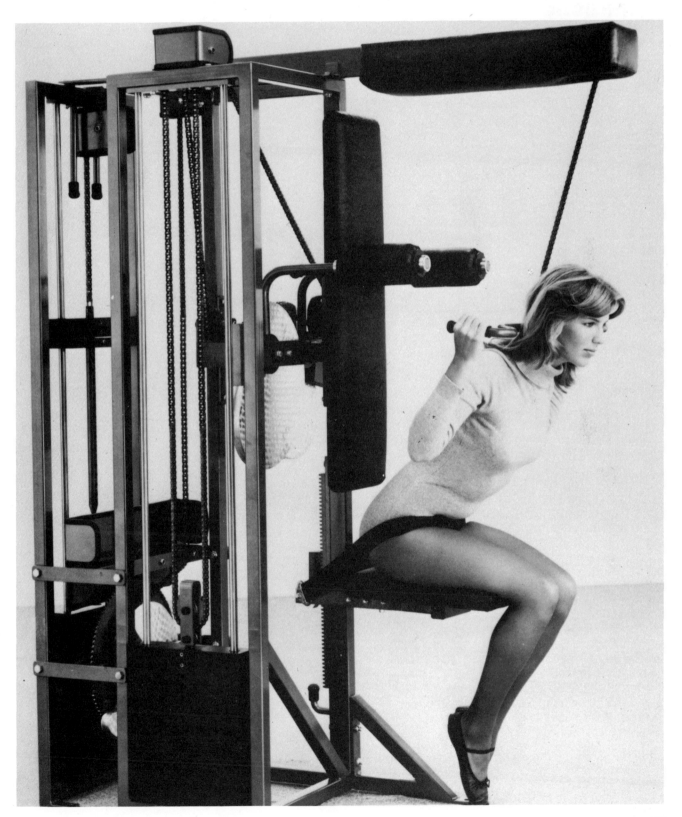

Gymnastics

In bygone days, when you attended a "gym" class at school or college, you worked out in gymnastics: the parallel bars, the vaulting horse, the horizontal bar, and tumbling. Then the Olympic Games demonstrated to an astonished world that gymnastic competition was one of the most graceful, demanding, and skilled precision sports in the whole Olympic pantheon. Today, gymnastic exercises will afford any athlete sound training in mobility, balance, and strength. They're also good warm-up exercises. With the exception of tumbling, equipment is required.

The big, expensive variable-resistance machines are not for the athlete who must do some or a great deal of his fitness training at home, but there is a small variety of inexpensive devices that can be of substantial benefit.

A stationary bicycle is a must if you don't have a place to run outdoors. Rope jumping is another alternative to running. A treadmill serves the same purpose, but—like cycling on a stationary bicycle or jumping in place—it can be terribly boring. The treadmill consists of a series of rollers that give you the effect of running without moving out of a circumscribed area; try to get one with a mileage meter and, if possible, a pulse meter. It is an excellent cardiovascular and respiratory training adjunct.

The rowing machine combines muscle-building and endurance conditioning for arms and legs alike. Some models also have an adjustable resistance arrangement so that you can step up the effort required.

Muscle "expanders" consisting of springs or rubber cords attached to handles will help develop the arm, shoulder, and chest muscles. A similar device known as a bullworker can be used with both arms and legs.

A wide variety of hand and grip strengtheners can be found in athletic stores, but as good a device as any for this purpose is a reasonably firm rubber ball (or two) for developing fingers, hands, and forearms.

For chinning, an adjustable horizontal bar can be set in a doorway. Experience will teach you that these devices are not infallibly secure; a good mat beneath the bar is recommended.

The chief item of equipment for competitive fitness is the human body, driven and abetted by motivation and discipline.

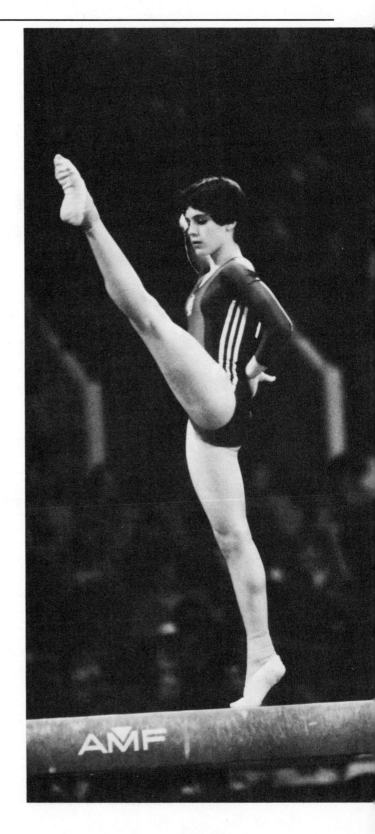

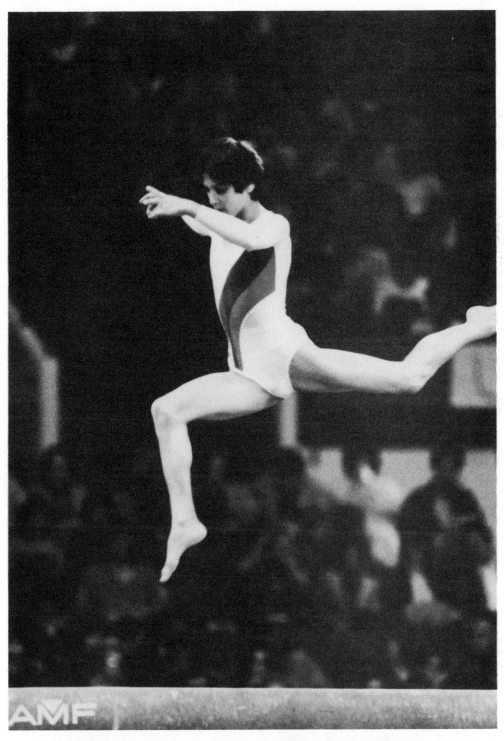

*My advice to a girl who wants to get into gymnastics is to join a group and start taking class lessons by the time she is seven.
—Johnny Hamilton, coach, artistic gymnastics team*

CHAPTER IV: FITNESS PROGRAM FOR THE COMPETITIVE MALE

From warm-ups through stretching and cardiovascular strengthening into body molding, the following synthesis of Olympic training exercises is programmed for the adult male who wants better physical capacity and is willing to work for it.

There are 32 exercises divided into three groups according to the part of the body being developed. The exercises are designed to create a basic level that provides the serious sportsman with a weekly routine. The exercise schedule is based on four sessions a week, though it can be reduced to three if time or facilities are limited. Each of the exercises is numbered: Do odd-numbered exercises on days 1 and 3 of your four-day exercise schedule and do the even-numbered exercises on days 2 and 4.

Each exercise has the number of sets and repetitions to be included in the Basic program. (A set is a group of repetitions; a repetition is the performance of an exercise from start to finish.) Also included are the added sets and repetitions that lift the program to the Improved and then to the Advanced stages of fitness. In a period of 10 to 12 weeks, the athlete who seeks ultimate conditioning will be working out at the Advanced level and will be devoting approximately 70 minutes a day, four days a week. In no case should your workout exceed an hour and a half, including warm-up.

The athlete who seeks strength and flexibility and improved endurance but does not have the time, desire, or perhaps the physical capacity to achieve maximum conditioning can remain at the Basic level or proceed at his own pace to the Improved stage.

Each body has its own capabilities and its own limitations. In all of these exercises, it is important to remember the principle of *overload*. No two athletes have the exact same muscle development. Some exercises will be easier for one and more difficult for another. Variations in sets and repetitions should be dictated by your physical capabilities. The guideline is: Push yourself to the utmost but no farther. If you cannot do all the repetitions called for, do as many as you can and then go on to the next exercise, always staying in sequence. When you have finished the routine, rest for a short period, drink water or diluted fruit juice if you're thirsty, and then go back and try to finish the uncompleted exercises. If you miss an exercise schedule, try to perform the stretching exercises and do some aerobic activity. So far as possible, stretching and aerobics should be part of your daily lifestyle.

Remember: You are competitive, which is why you are reading this. Compete with yourself. Try to reach the Improved level. Then reach for the Advanced. Your reward will be improved performance by an athlete with a better body in better condition (as your opponents may well find out themselves).

A helpful rule of thumb in working out: By week 4, you should be approaching the Improved level. By week 10, you'll be approaching the Advanced—if that is your goal.

Warm-up

Warm-up is just what the name implies: It is a short period—up to fifteen minutes—of easy movement intended to warm the muscles, increase the blood circulation, and expand respiration. The warm-up sends oxygen through the blood at a quicker pace. Muscles become more flexible, helping to prevent injury that may come from sudden effort—the muscles most affected and most susceptible to injury not being the contracting muscles, which power your movements, but the opposing, relaxing muscles, which may be forced to expand too rapidly too suddenly.

The warm-up must *immediately precede* vigorous action. Cool off between the warm-up and the event, and you're in worse shape than with no warm-up at all.

You will want to modify your warm-up regimen for your particular sport or specialty if you are a team athlete. If you are simply a competitive male, choose from among the following exercises to suit yourself. Remember that the purpose is to warm the muscles, to increase the blood flow, and not to push yourself to a level of intense exertion.

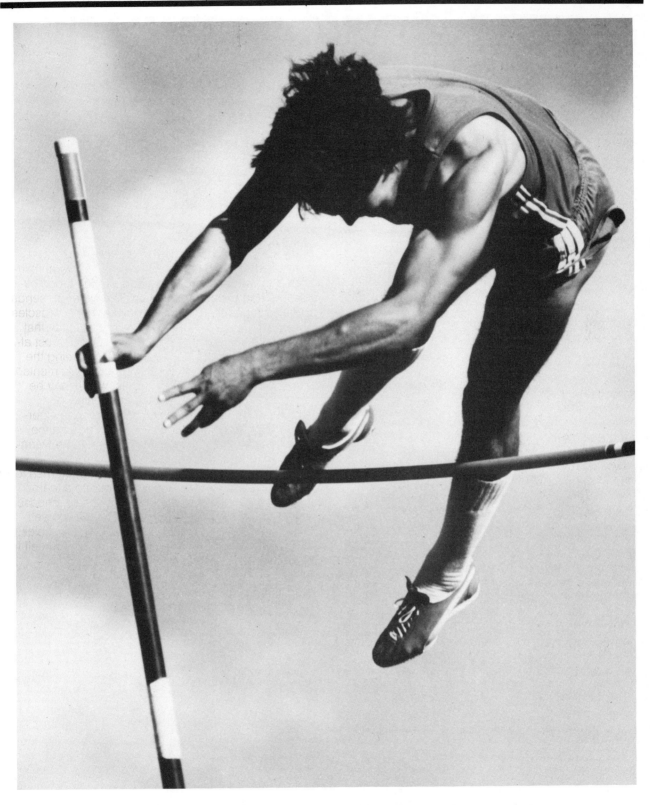

A good warm-up should stretch all the major muscles of the body then isolate those that are central to your sport for special emphasis. But you must warm up all the muscles in rotation because they all have to function together.
  —Steve Hornor, soccer trainer

1/
BEND DOWNS

Standing with feet together and arms at your sides,
bend over from the waist and reach toward your ankles, then your toes. Up to 10 repetitions

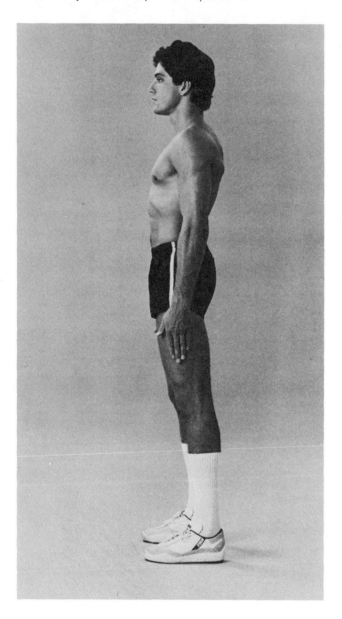 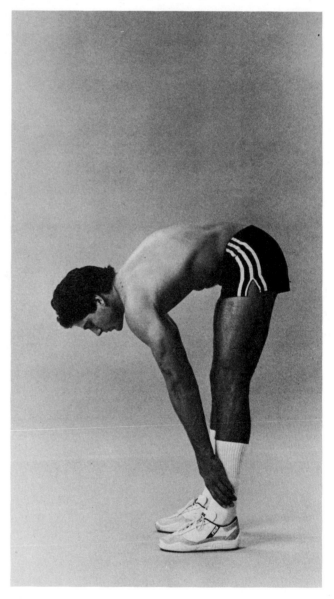

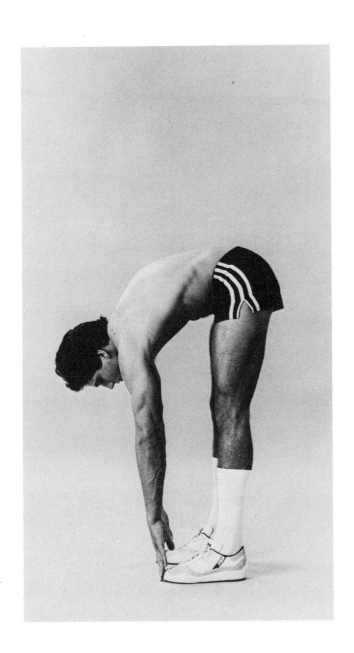

2/
SQUAT BOUNCE

With your left leg straight behind you, squat on your right leg with hands pointing forward, palms on the floor. Bounce up and change positions of your right and left legs. Up to 12 repetitions

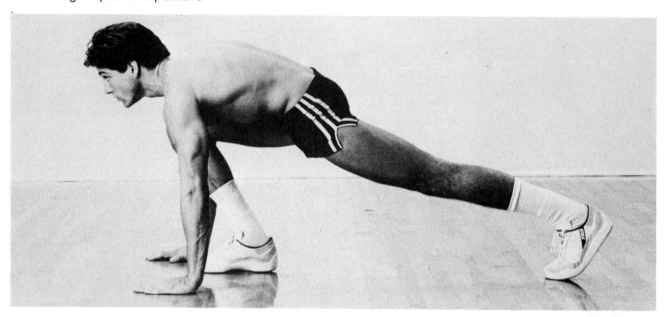

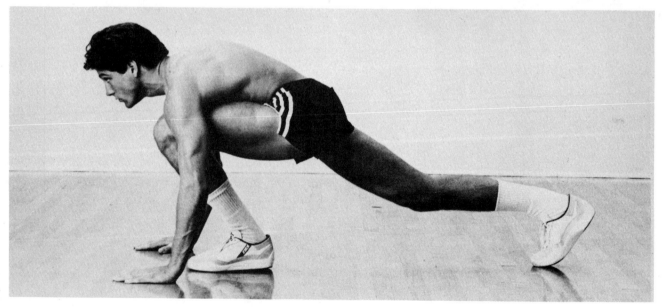

3/
FLOOR STRETCH

Sit on the floor, legs apart and stretched out in front of
you, hands on your knees. Bend from the waist and,
with your head down, place your hands on the floor
as far in front of you as possible. Up to 12 repetitions

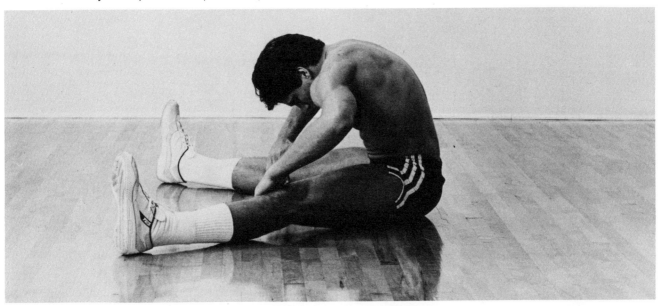

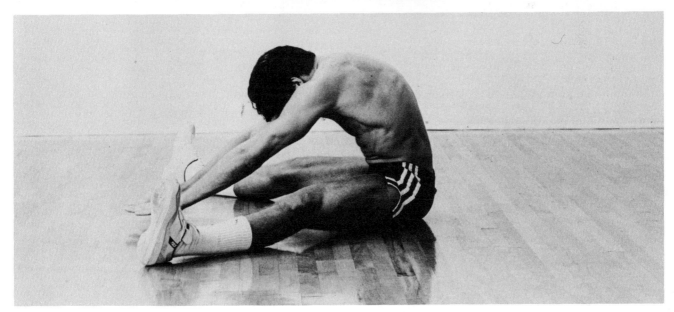

4/
SCISSORS

Lie on your right side with your right arm extended on the floor above your head, your left arm resting on side or used for balance. Lift your left leg about 2 feet off the floor and lower it. Up to 12 repetitions

Same exercise for your right leg. Up to 12 repetitions

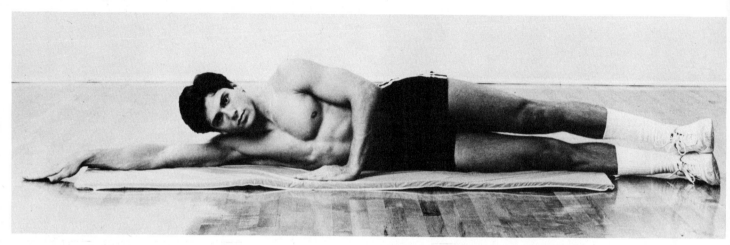

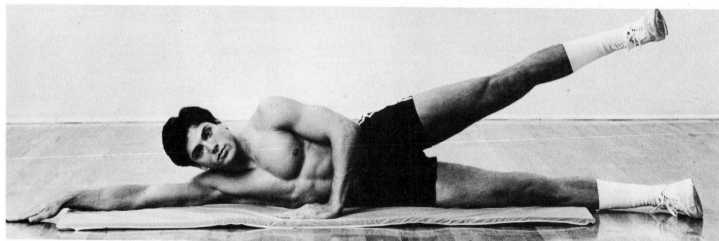

5/
RUN AND JUMPS

Run in place to a count of 60, lifting each foot at least 4 inches off the ground. Then do 10 saddle hops or jumping jacks (stand erect, hands at sides, feet to-gether; raise hands straight above your head to clap together and jump legs about two feet apart to a straddle position. Return to first position.).

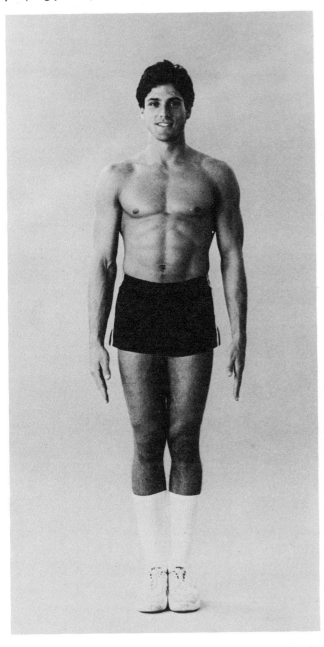
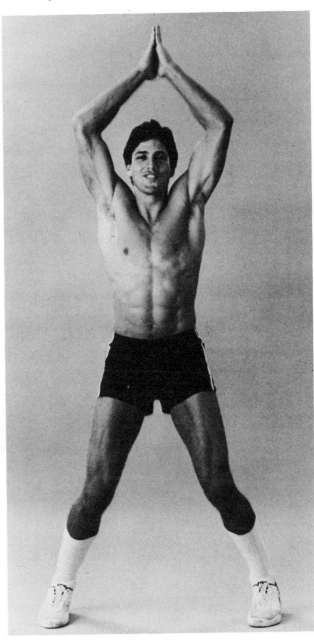

6/
FORWARD CURL

Lie on your back, legs together, knees bent, and arms stretched above your head. Raise your trunk to a sitting position, then slide your hands forward along your knees until they are stretched out in front of you. 5 repetitions

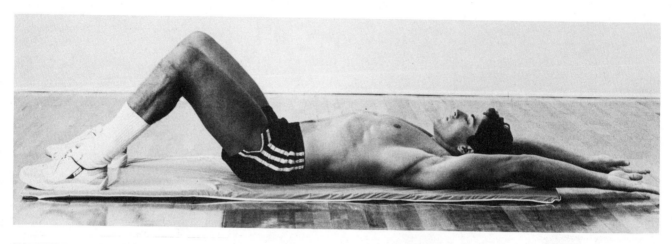

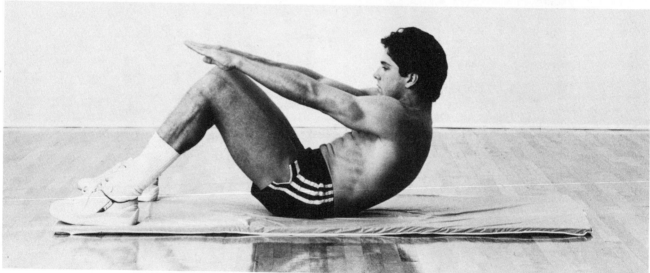

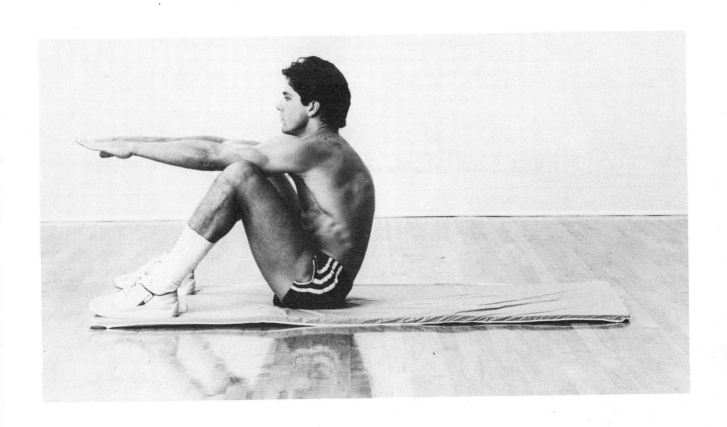

Stretching

Muscle flexibility is as vital to top performance as strength and endurance. Muscles and tendons inevitably shorten when not in active use. Flexibility exercises should be a daily routine, even if only for a few minutes. The term "muscle-bound" refers to muscles that are too taut. A weight lifter who develops his biceps and neglects his triceps suffers this fate, usually recognizable by his carrying his muscular arms in a slightly bent position. Anyone can become muscle-bound though, so from the following choose those stretching routines that best fit your sport.

NOTE: All of these stretching exercises should be done slowly and gracefully. Stretching and warm-ups are intended to loosen you up, not wear you out. Stretching exercises should be a daily routine. Before a game or event, warm up and stretch until you break a sweat.

1/
HAMSTRING LIMBER-UP

With legs together, stoop and place hands on the floor directly in front of you. Straighten legs, keeping hands on floor. Return to upright position. Hold for 15 seconds, 3 repetitions.

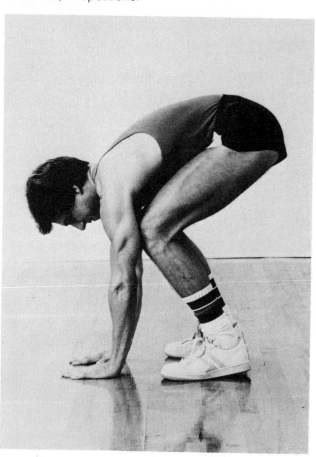
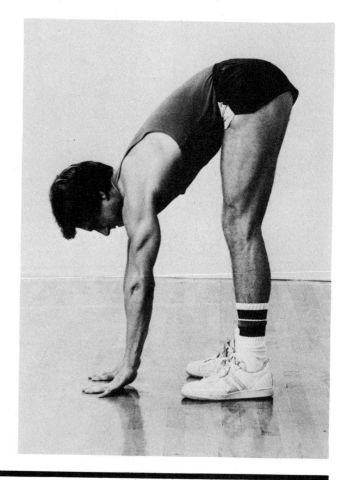

2/
ACHILLES' TENDON

Stand about 3 feet from a wall, feet slightly apart. Place your hands flat on the wall, directly in front of your shoulders, arms stiff. Now bend elbows and let your head come to the wall, keeping feet flat on the ground. Hold for 15 seconds, 3 repetitions.

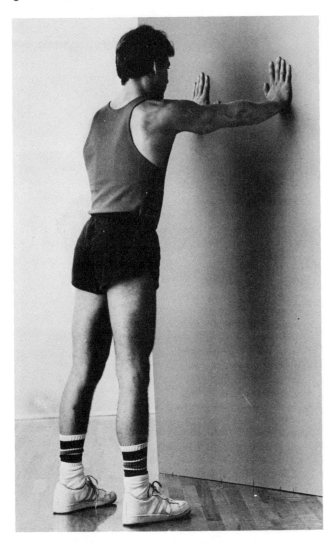
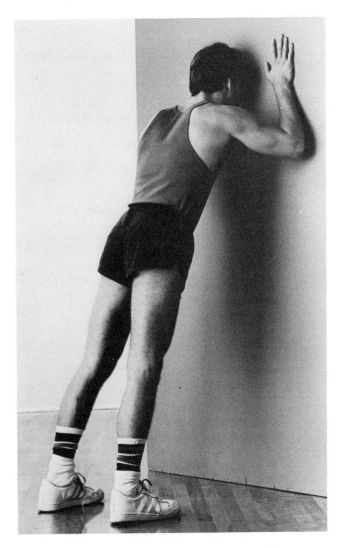

3/
SIDE STRETCHER

The psoas is the muscle that links the back, hip, and thigh. It is one of the most important muscles of the body to keep limber. In this stretch, lie on your back and pull each knee to your forehead. Hold for 15 seconds, 3 repetitions.

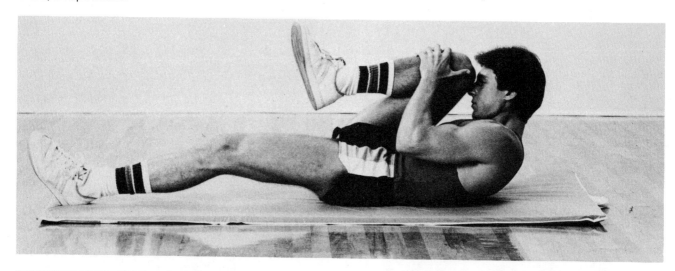

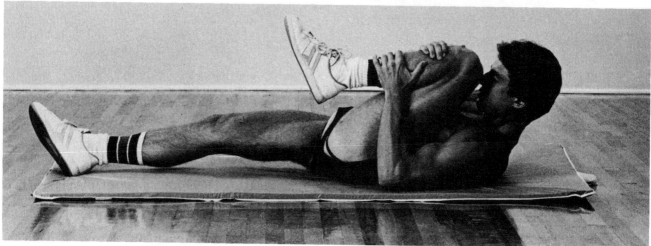

4/
SPINE CURL

Lying on your back with your knees bent and raised, arms crossed over the chest, raise your head as high and as far forward as you can. Return to supine position. Hold for 15 seconds, 3 repetitions.

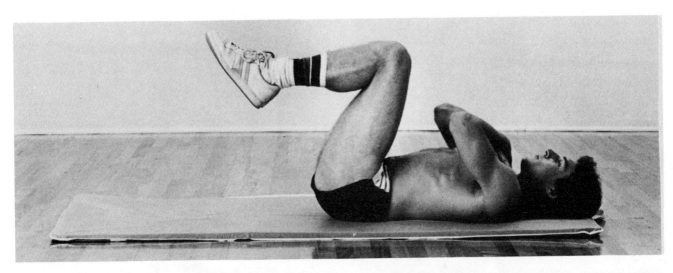

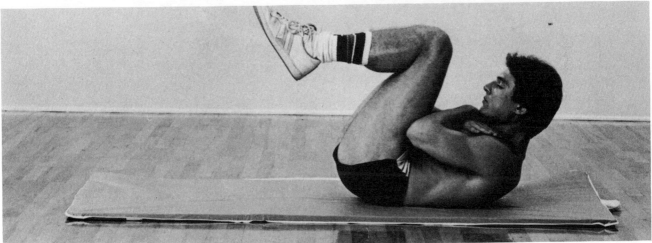

5/
TORSO TWIST

Stand with arms extended horizontally. Slowly twist
your body first to the left and then to the right as far
as you can. Keep head turned in a direction opposite
to the twist. Continue for 30 seconds.

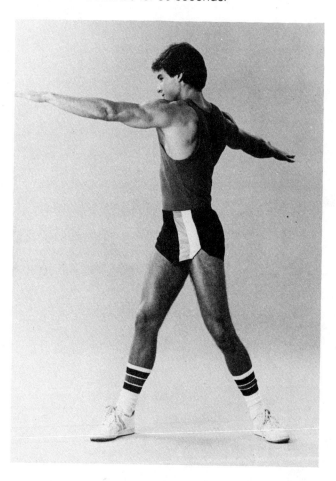 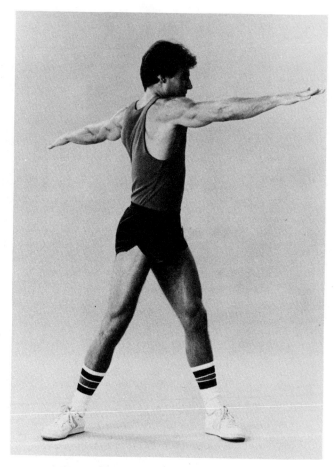

6/
WINDMILLS

With left arm extended horizontally forward and right
arm backward, describe large, slow, circular windmill
rotations. Continue for 30 seconds.

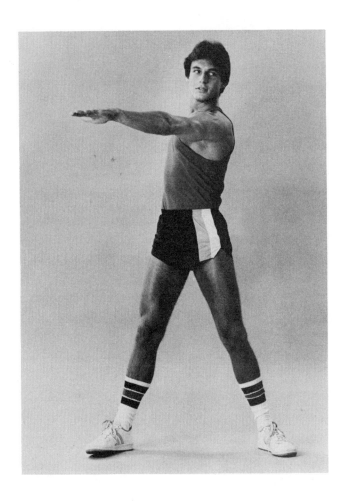
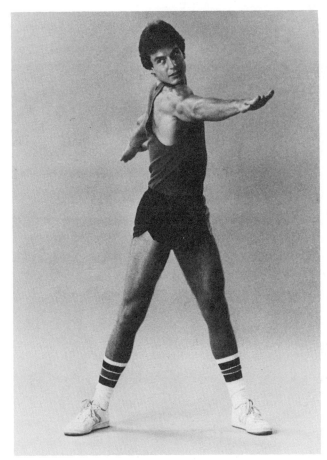

7/
ADDUCTOR FLEX

Limbering the groin muscles. Lie on your back, knees bent, feet together. Let the knees fall outward as far as they will go. Place hands on inside of knees and press your legs apart, keeping feet together. Hold 10 seconds, relax 5 seconds, and repeat.

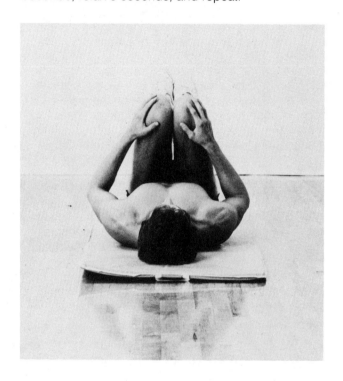 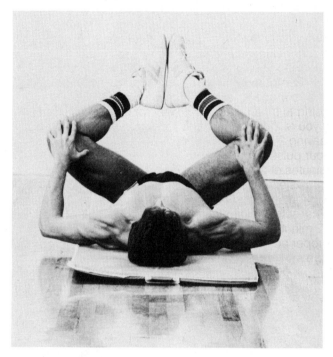

Aerobic Conditioning

You're an athlete. You come to this program in reasonably good condition. What you're aiming for is a tougher kind of conditioning, one that will fit you for competition. You know that endurance is a key factor in all active sports and that to achieve your maximum endurance you must train your cardio-respiratory system to supply the maximum fuel and oxygen to your muscles during competition.

The best exercises for building up the heart, blood vessels, and lungs are running (or running in place), bicycling, swimming, rope skipping, and—in heavy doses—aerobic dancing. How can you tell if you're getting full benefit from your workout? By checking your pulse rate after your aerobic exercise.

Remember the formula: 220 beats a minute minus your age times 70 percent. (Eventually, we're going to try to build that pulse rate up to 80 percent.) If you're 20 years old, subtract that age from 220, leaving 200, of which 70 percent is 140. That's what your pulse rate should be after 15, 20, or more minutes of aerobic exercise.

As a serious athlete, you should plan on four workouts a week. Dr. Ken Cooper, the father of aerobics, sets a minimum running schedule of 1½ miles in 12 minutes or less, four days a week, to achieve proper aerobic conditioning. If you prefer riding a bike, make sure that you cover 3 miles in 11½

minutes, twice a day, four days a week. For those who use a stationary bike, set up a clock where you can watch it and adjust your speed so that you cover the required 3 miles in the indicated 11½ minutes.

For those occasions when you have no facilities for running, swimming, or biking, no treadmill and no rowing machine, there still remain running in place and rope skipping. The latter is more interesting, and a considerable amount of expertise can be developed. The usual children's rope skip is two bounces for every spin of the rope. Gradually improve your skill to one bounce for each rope turn. Then work up to alternating your feet, crossing your hands, and even trying to make two or three turns of the rope on one bounce.

If you must do your jogging on asphalt, and you have a stride that comes down hard, jolting your spine, a trick that many joggers use is to go into a slight Groucho Marx-type crouch with bent knees. This enables you to run with your head and shoulders on a fairly level plane and eliminates the jouncing effect that can cause discomfort and even physical damage.

Before you continue your workout, replace the water you've lost. Do not add salt or any other substance to the water. The only alternative is fruit juice—which may be diluted—but water is quite adequate, at the rate of a glass for every 15 minutes of aerobic exercise.

After six to eight weeks of inactivity, you have lost virtually all of your aerobic conditioning.
—Dr. Richard Stedman, physician to Olympic ski and ice hockey teams

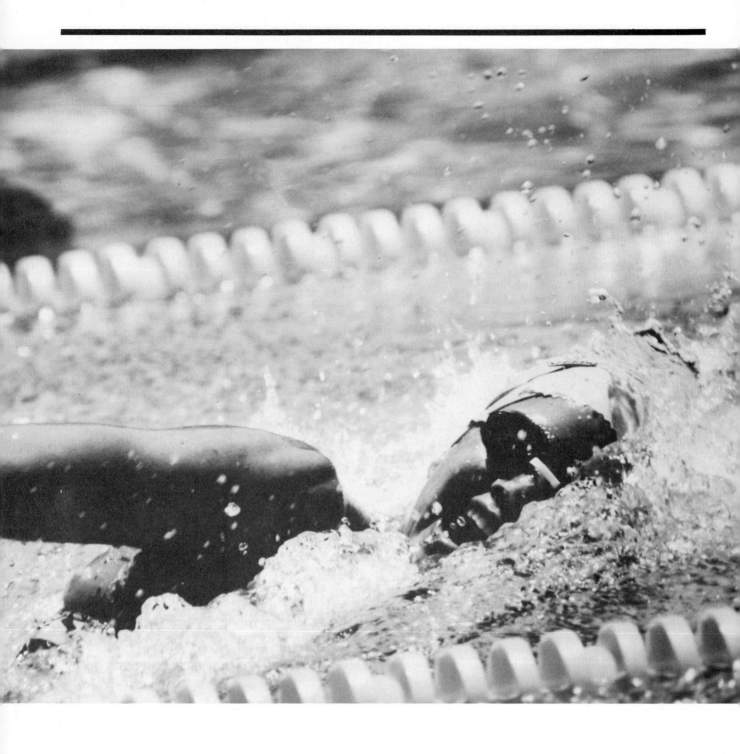

Sometimes I swim fast, and I can't understand why. But it's because I had hard training before.
—Vladimir Slanikov, gold medalist, 400- and 1500-meter freestyle 1980 Olympic and world record holder

Exercises for the Competitive Male

The exercises are divided into three groups, according to the area of the body being developed: the upper body, the mid body, the lower body. Remember that the sets and repetitions listed in these exercises are goals, not immediate minimums. Do as many as you can until you start hurting. Then go on to the next exercise.

The Upper Body

The human shoulder is beautifully designed. The shoulder blade, called the scapula, ends in a socket. Into this socket, forming a ball joint, fits the round knob at the upper end of the humerus, the bone behind the biceps. The ball joint allows a wide range of motion to the arm, and the muscles and tendons that control these movements are among the most important in the body. The exercises for the arms and shoulders begin with a classic muscle-building exercise—the push-up.

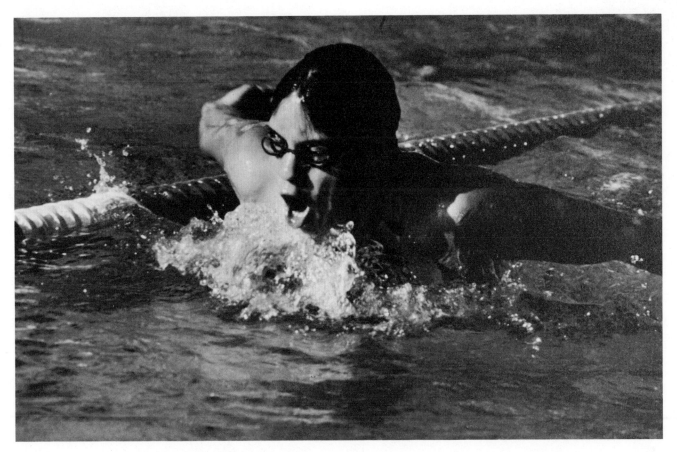

1/
PUSH-UPS

With your weight on your hands and toes and your body straight and firm from ankles to head, push up from the ground until your arms are straight. Then let down until your chest touches. Don't let down too fast. Sports medicine is placing new emphasis on *negative* exercise; that is, exercise that is performed working with gravity rather than against it. This is an extremely important aspect of strength building.

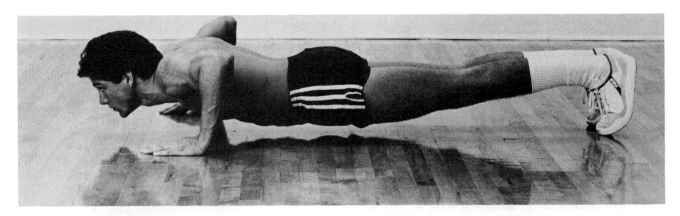

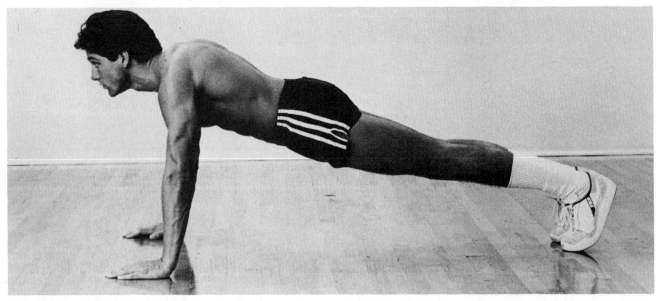

DAYS 1, 3

Basic:	2 sets of 10 repetitions
Improved:	3 sets of 15 repetitions
Advanced:	4 sets of 20 repetitions

2/
PUMP-UPS

Using 3 chairs, one on either side of you and one about 4 feet in front of you, place your palms on the side chairs and your heels on the front chair so that the body forms a right angle. Now ease yourself down almost to the floor and then pump back up.

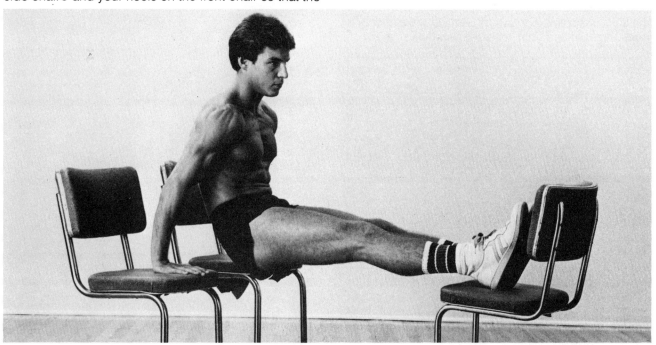

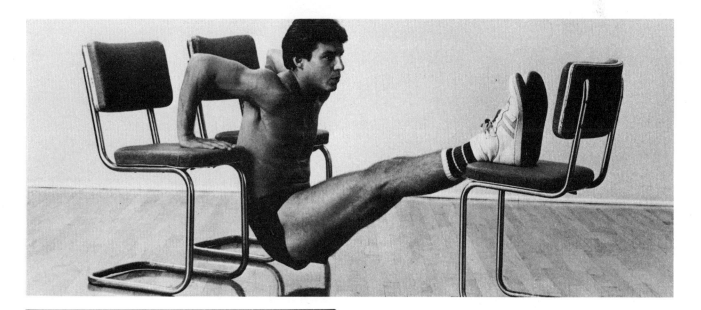

DAYS 2, 4

Basic:	3 sets of 20 repetitions
Improved:	4 sets of 22 repetitions
Advanced:	5 sets of 24 repetitions

3/
CHIN-UPS

Use a gym chinning bar or one that can be installed in a doorway of your home. Home bars sometimes slip. Keep a mat below or install the round metal supports that are used with clothes poles in closets. Palms can face away or toward you. Pull your chin above the pole and then ease yourself down.

DAYS 1, 3

Basic:	3 sets of 5 repetitions
Improved:	5 sets of 12 repetitions
Advanced:	6 sets of 15 repetitions

4/
FRENCH CURL

In a standing position, feet apart and firmly planted on the floor, bring a barbell to a position behind your neck with your elbows pointing upward. Raise the barbell until your elbows and arms are straight. Lower the barbell to your shoulders slowly. Start with 5 pound weights and increase steadily as you build muscle.

Perform the same exercise but with elbows pointing downward and palms facing up. Grip on the barbell should be wider for this one. 2 sets of 5 repetitions

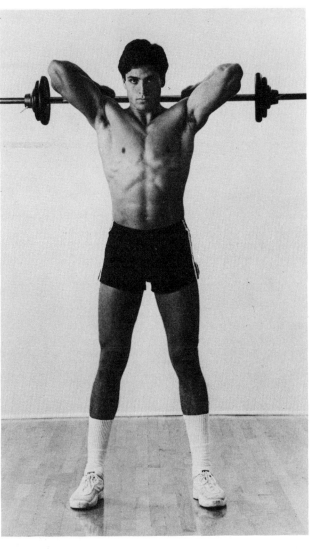

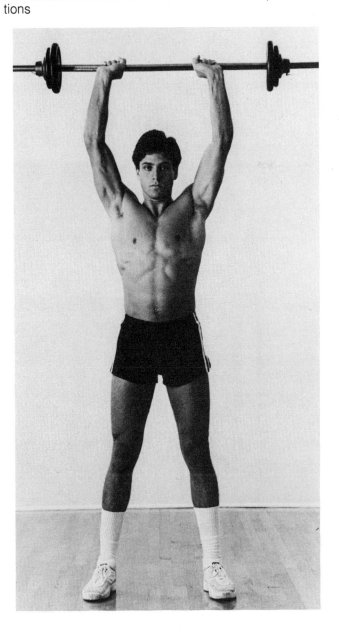

DAYS 2, 4

Basic:	4 sets of 5 repetitions
Improved:	6 sets of 10 repetitions
Advanced:	6 sets of 12 repetitions

5/
WRIST CURL

Sit on a chair or bench with wrists over your knees, palms up, holding barbell by fingers. Bend wrists up and then return. Same exercise with palms facing down. 2 sets of 10 repetitions

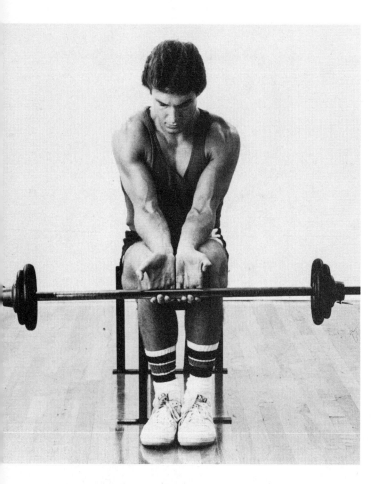 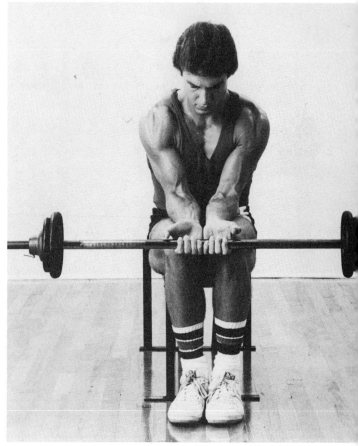

DAYS 1, 3

Basic:	5 sets of 12 repetitions
Improved:	6 sets of 12 repetitions
Advanced:	6 sets of 12 repetitions

6/
BENCH PRESS

Although there are many types of presses of great value to muscle building, avoid standing presses without instructor or trainer guidance because of the possible danger of back strain. Lie on a bench with feet flat on the ground and raise and lower the barbell over your chest. Dumbbells may be used instead of the barbell.

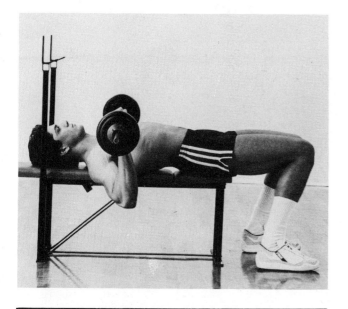

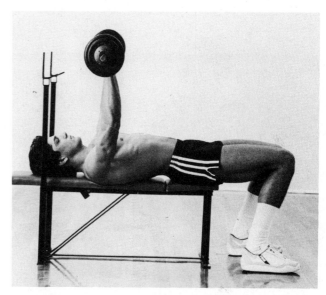

DAYS 2, 4

Basic:	5 sets of 5 repetitions
Improved:	8 sets of 9 repetitions
Advanced:	8 sets of 10 repetitions

7/
BICEPS CURL

Hold barbell palms up with elbows at your sides and forearms extended forward. Bring the barbell to your chest and then return slowly. Return slowly. Remember the negative, or return, part of the exercise is as important as the positive.

The exercise can also be performed with dumbbells.

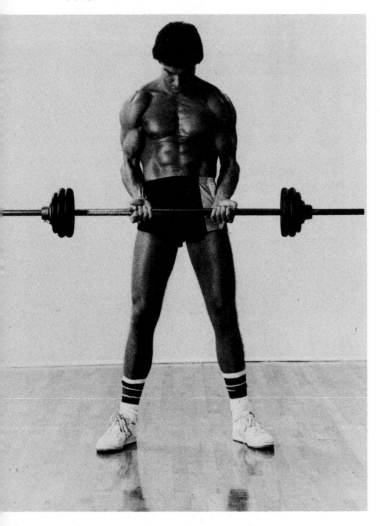 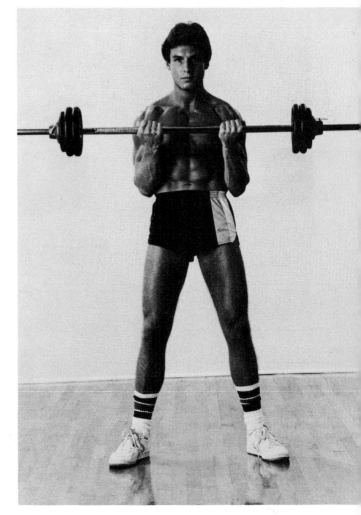

DAYS 1, 3

Basic:	5 sets of 10 repetitions
Improved:	8 sets of 12 repetitions
Advanced:	9 sets of 12 repetitions

8/
BUTTERFLY SWING

Lying back flat on a bench with feet on the ground, extend arms horizontally, holding dumbbells. Raise arms above your body until the dumbbells almost meet. Keep arms slightly bent.

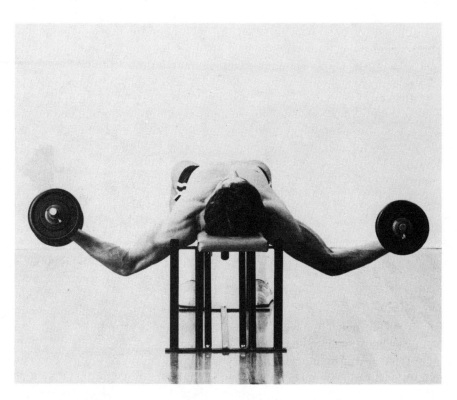 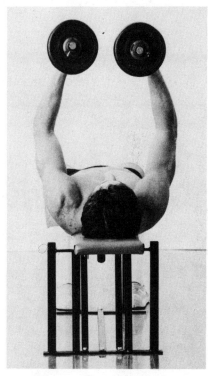

DAYS 2, 4

Basic:	3 sets of 10 repetitions
Improved:	5 sets of 15 repetitions
Advanced:	5 sets of 15 repetitions

9/
BALL CLUTCH

Using a rubber ball (about the size of a racquetball), squeeze slowly for about 3 seconds and hold. Then release and repeat. (A grip developer with springs may be used instead of the ball.)

DAYS 1, 3	
Basic:	4 sets of 12 repetitions
Improved:	7 sets of 12 repetitions
Advanced:	8 sets of 12 repetitions

10/
TOWEL WRING

Using a rolled-up bath towel, hold it with hands about shoulder-width apart. Wring the towel as hard as you can. Unwring and repeat.

DAYS 2, 4	
Basic:	2 sets of 5 repetitions
Improved:	5 sets of 8 repetitions
Advanced:	5 sets of 10 repetitions

The Mid Body

The mid body is where it all comes together. The mid-body muscles do not perform feats of speed and endurance like the legs or exhibit the power and skill of the arms, but they are the fulcrum on which you must balance your competitive achievements. We start with a classic exercise for the abdominal muscles—bent-knee sit-ups.

1/
BENT-KNEE SIT-UPS

Lying on your back with your hands clasped behind your head, raise your knees until they form a right angle. You may put your feet under a bureau, desk, bookcase, or fixed rod, or you may simply rest them on the ground. Rise to an upright sitting position and then slowly lower your head and back to the ground.

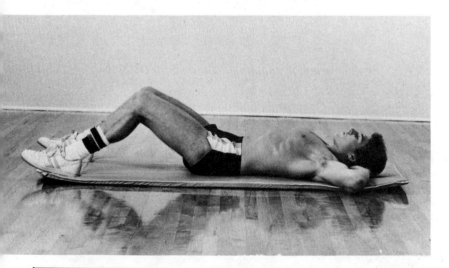 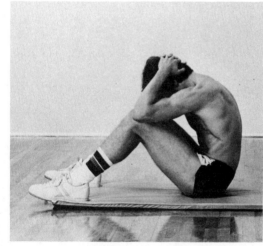

DAYS 1, 3

Basic:	4 sets of 10 repetitions
Improved:	5 sets of 15 repetitions
Advanced:	5 sets of 18 repetitions

2/
LEG LIFTS

Lying on the floor with your hands either beside your thighs or above your head grasping a firm, fixed object, raise your legs to a vertical position. Then lower slowly. This again is essentially a negative exercise, so emphasize the slow return of your legs to the floor.

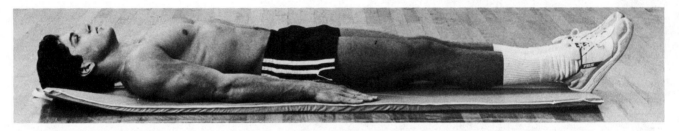

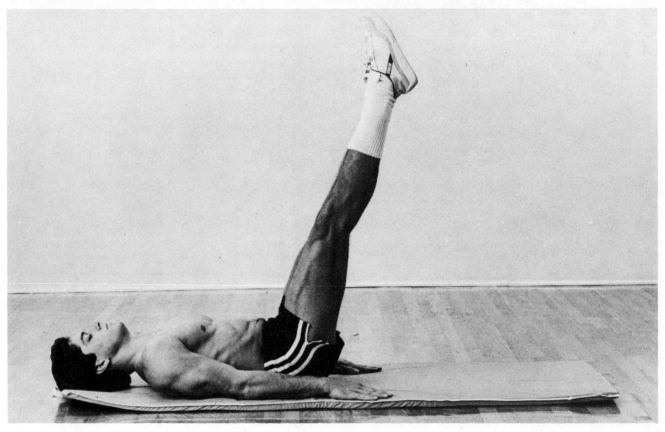

DAYS 2, 4

Basic:	2 sets of 20 repetitions
Improved:	1 set of 40 repetitions
Advanced:	1 set of 50 repetitions

3/
DUMBBELL LIFTS

Holding a dumbbell in each hand with feet firmly planted on the ground, lift first one, then the other, high above your head, at the same time dropping the opposing arm so that your body arches toward the down-side dumbbell.

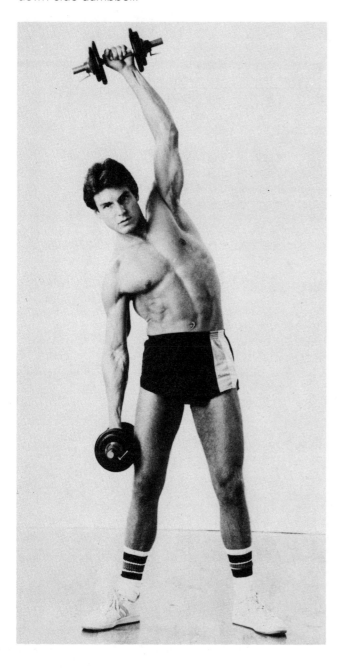 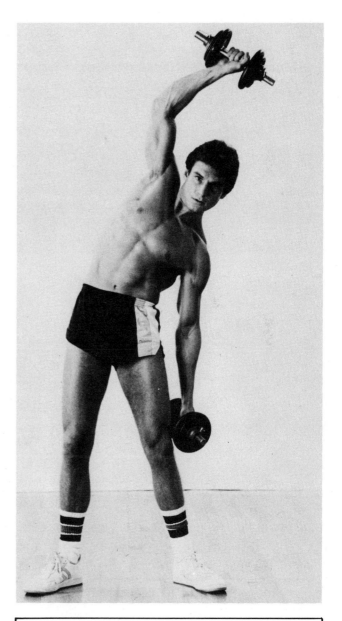

DAYS 1, 3

Basic:	2 sets of 25 repetitions
Improved:	2 sets of 30 repetitions
Advanced:	2 sets of 35 repetitions

4/
FOOT LIFTS

Lying on your back, hands under your head, raise your legs about 10 inches off the ground. Keep your legs straight and feet together. Hold feet raised for 10 seconds, then lower. Excellent for the psoas muscles.

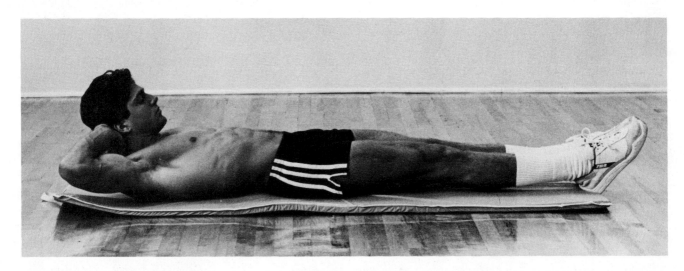

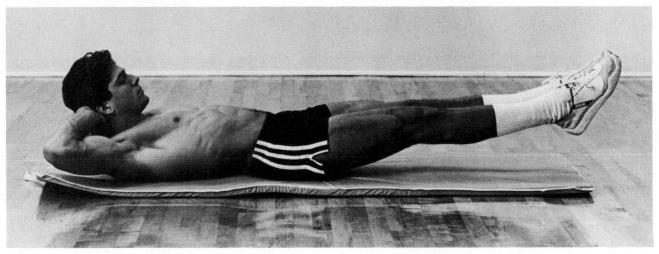

DAYS 2, 4

Basic:	1 set of 30 repetitions
Improved:	1 set of 40 repetitions
Advanced:	2 sets of 30 repetitions

5/
LIFT-OFFS

Lying prone (face down) with a pillow under your hips and abdomen and your feet firmly anchored under a desk or bureau (or with someone holding them firmly to the floor), clasp your hands behind your neck and lift your head, chest, and shoulders off the ground. Hold for 10 seconds, then lower.

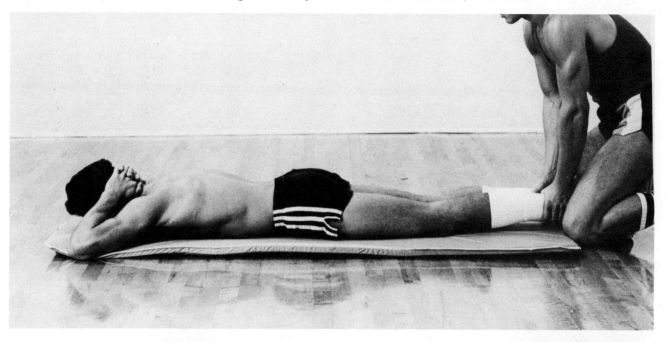

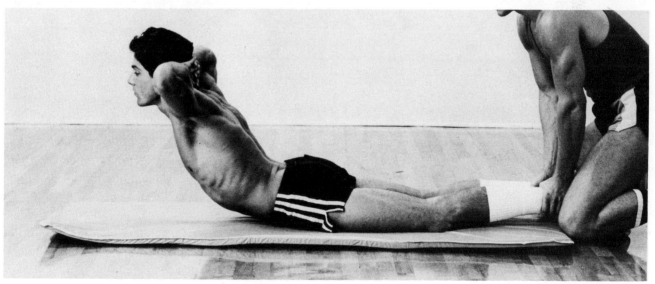

DAYS 1, 3	
Basic:	3 sets of 20 repetitions
Improved:	4 sets of 25 repetitions
Advanced:	4 sets of 25 repetitions

6/
ROUND-UP TWIST

Stand and lock your hands high above your head, bending slightly backward. From the waist, bend all the way to the right, around, touching the ground in front of you, and then up on the left side. Reverse the direction and repeat.

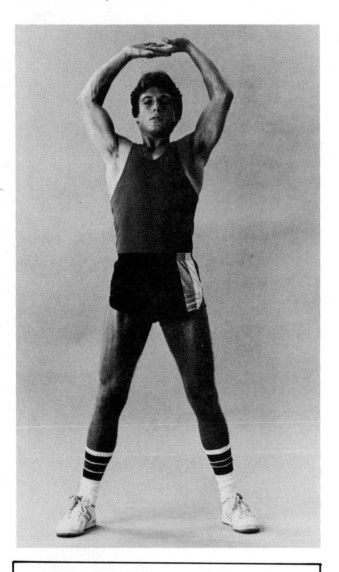 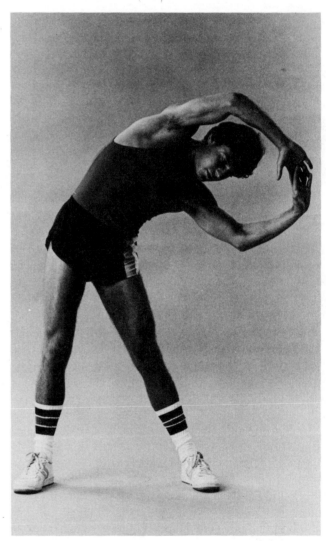

DAYS 2, 4

Basic:	2 sets of 12 repetitions
Improved:	2 sets of 20 repetitions
Advanced:	3 sets of 15 repetitions

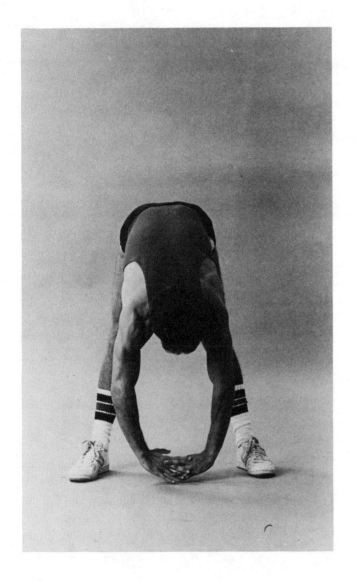

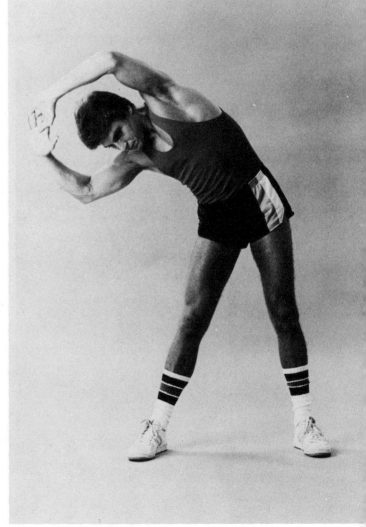

7/
TORSO TORSION

Place your left foot on a chair. Clasp your hands high above your head. Bend forward with clasped hands and touch your left toe. Then down and touch your right toe, then up and out on your right side, arms still straight. Repeat with the opposite foot on the chair.

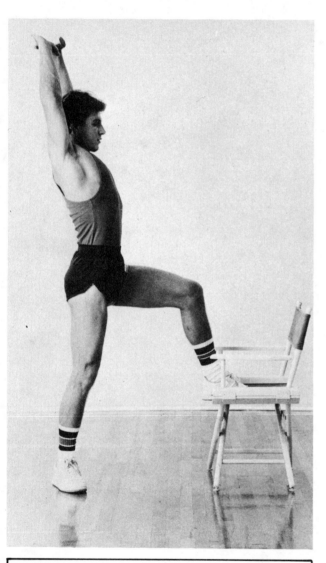
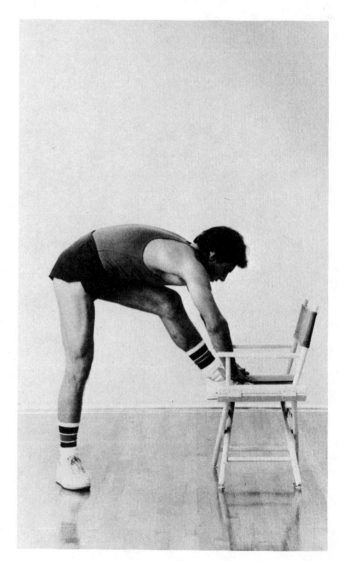

DAYS 1, 3	
Basic:	2 sets of 10 repetitions
Improved:	3 sets of 12 repetitions
Advanced:	3 sets of 12 repetitions

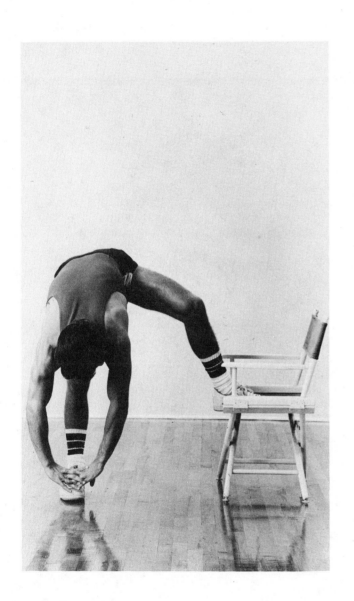

8/
PUNTING PRACTICE

Hold your arm straight out in front of you, and, rising slightly on the ball of your left foot, swing your right foot back and then up to touch your right hand. Repeat with the opposite foot.

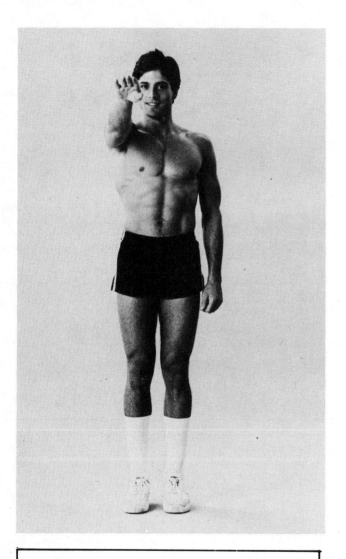 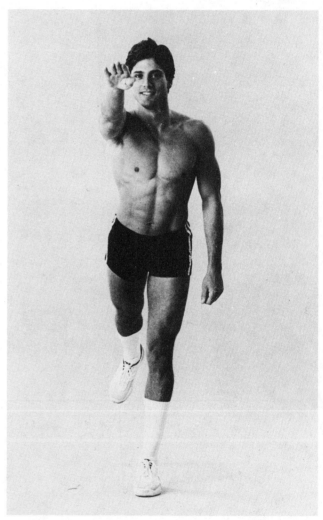

DAYS 2, 4

Basic:	2 sets of 7 repetitions
Improved:	3 sets of 8 repetitions
Advanced:	3 sets of 10 repetitions

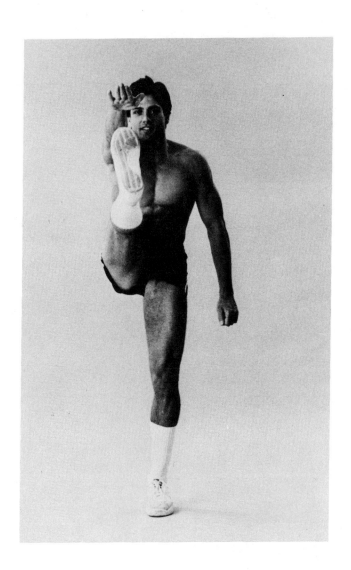

9/
WEIGHT SWING

With your feet well apart, hold a dumbbell with both hands high above your head. First swing it in a wide circle in front of you. Next swing it forward and down between your legs, bending and pushing the weight as far aft as possible with your head about at knee level. Alternate the swing to the right and left.

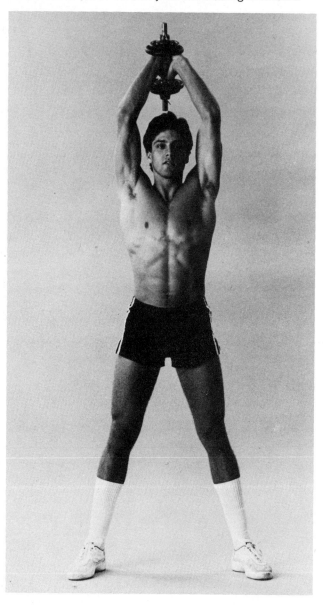 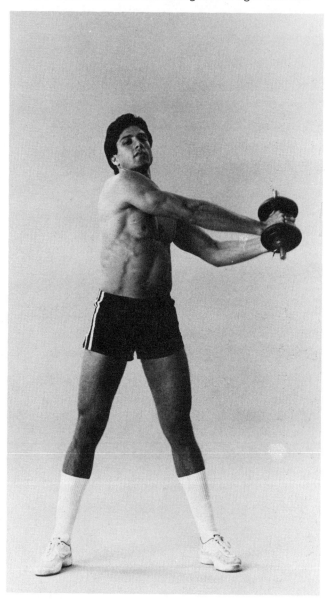

DAYS 1, 3	
Basic:	3 sets of 12 repetitions
Improved:	3 sets of 18 repetitions
Advanced:	3 sets of 20 repetitions

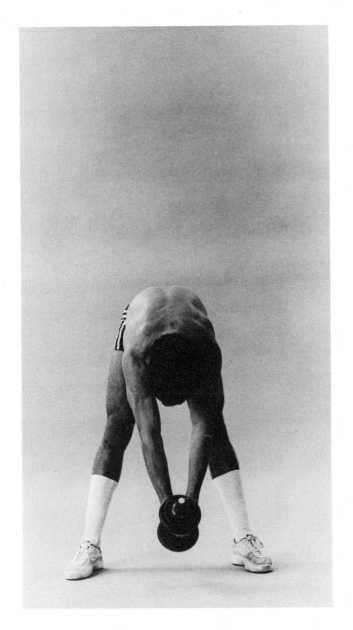 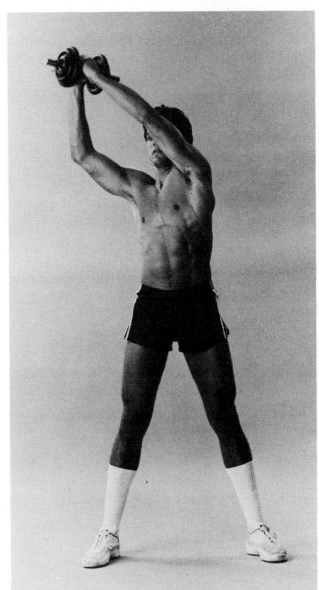

10/
TOWEL PULL

This is an excellent isometric exercise. With the end of a twisted bath towel in your right hand, place the opposite end under your right heel. Holding your left hand on your hip and knees straight, pull as hard as you can for 6 seconds. Repeat on the opposite side.

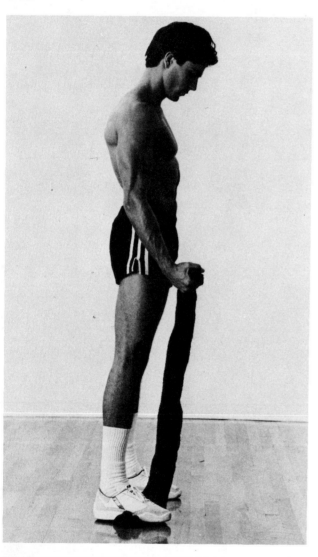
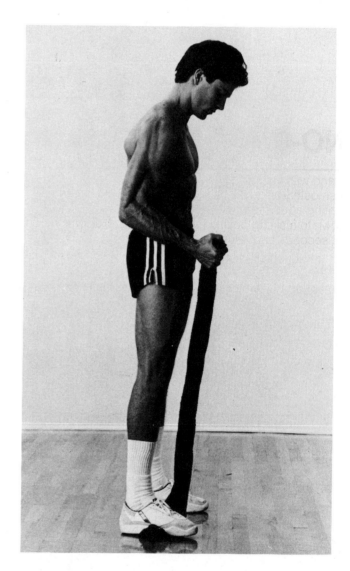

DAYS 2, 4

Basic:	2 sets of 8 repetitions
Improved:	3 sets of 15 repetitions
Advanced:	3 sets of 16 repetitions

The Lower Body

"If your calves and thighs ain't in shape, you haven't got a leg to stand on." No one remembers the coach who uttered that sage observation, but in sports, you can't argue his point. Literally and figuratively, your legs form the base on which you build. If you jog or skip rope or run in place in your aerobic exercises, you will be building up your calf and thigh muscles. The following exercises are specifically directed toward complementing and augmenting any running you do.

1/
NO-CHAIR SIT

Stand with your feet a little apart, about 10 inches from a smooth wall. Lean back until your upper body is resting against the wall. Now bend knees and slide down to a sitting position. Stay in sitting position for 15 seconds and return to upright.

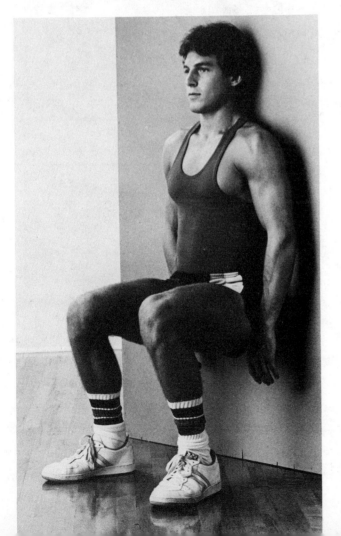

DAYS 1, 3	
Basic:	2 sets of 5 repetitions
Improved:	3 sets of 10 repetitions
Advanced:	3 sets of 12 repetitions

2/
HOP-UPS

With your feet slightly forward and arms behind you,
take a short hop forward, then a short hop back,
swinging your arms as you hop. Then swing your
arms over your head and jump as high as you can
with your head thrown back. This exercise goes well
with bouncy music as you maintain a steady rhythm:
forward, back, up, forward, back, up.

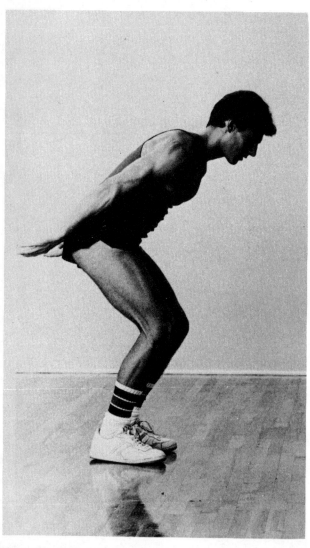 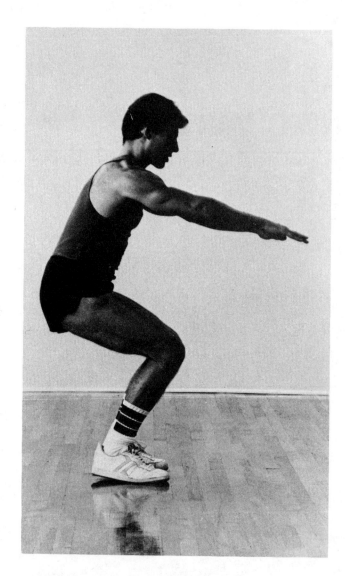

DAYS 2, 4

Basic:	3 sets of 20 repetitions
Improved:	3 sets of 30 repetitions
Advanced:	3 sets of 35 repetitions

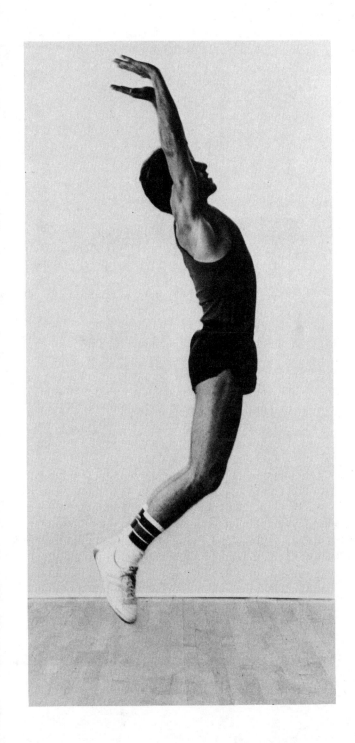

3/
KNEEBENDS

With hands on hips, drop to a half squat; that is, without resting the buttocks on the heels but rather with the thighs about parallel to the ground. Then rise to the erect position. Keep chin up.

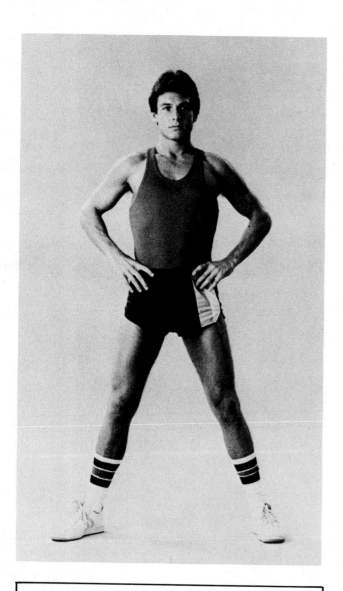

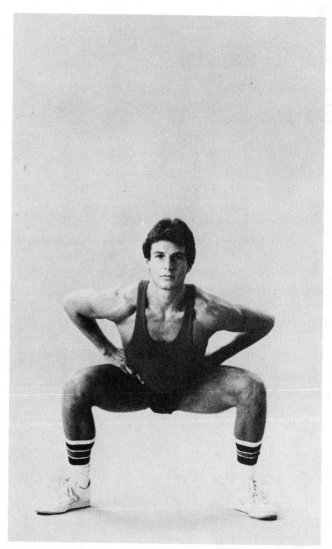

DAYS 1, 3

Basic:	2 sets of 25 repetitions
Improved:	3 sets of 25 repetitions
Advanced:	3 sets of 30 repetitions

4/
WEIGHTED KNEEBENDS

In this half-squat kneebend, you will carry the barbell across your shoulders, behind your head. This is an ultimate muscle builder since you can continue to increase the weights on the barbells as you build power. Check with a trainer as the weights grow heavier. You will want to set the barbell in place from a rack or have someone help you lift it onto your back.

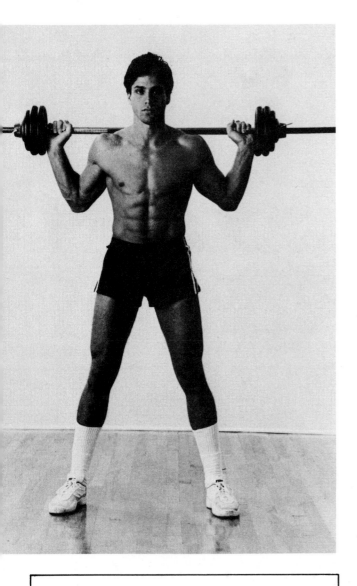

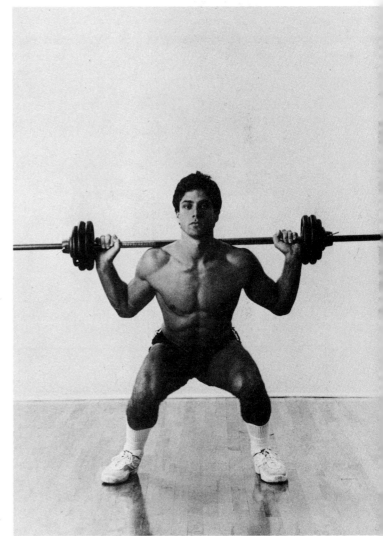

DAYS 2, 4

Basic:	3 sets of 12 repetitions
Improved:	3 sets of 20 repetitions
Advanced:	3 sets of 25 repetitions

5/
FOOT LIFTS

This exercise can be done with ankle weights or using an ordinary wastebasket. Sit on a chair, grasping the seat firmly with your hands. If you use weights, lift legs to a horizontal position. With a wastebasket, grasp it firmly between your feet and raise it till your legs are horizontal. Then set it back on the floor and repeat.

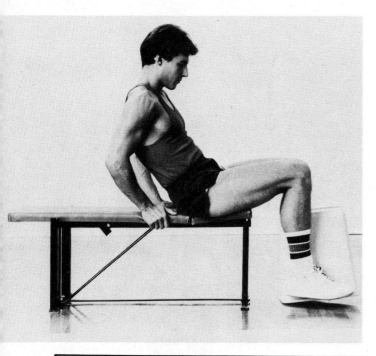 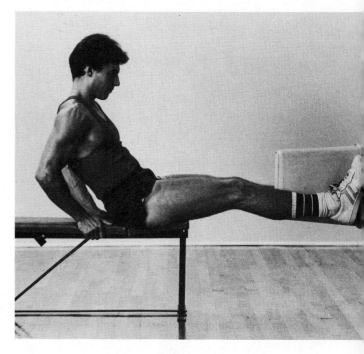

DAYS 1, 3	
Basic:	3 sets of 10 repetitions
Improved:	4 sets of 20 repetitions
Advanced:	4 sets of 25 repetitions

6/
HEEL DIPS

Stand on the balls of your feet on the edge of a step,
steadying yourself against the wall or bannister.
Your stance should be slightly pigeon-toed. Rise
up on your toes and then dip your heels below stair
level as far as they'll go. Repeat.

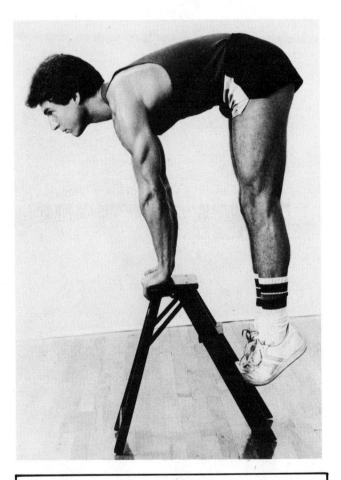 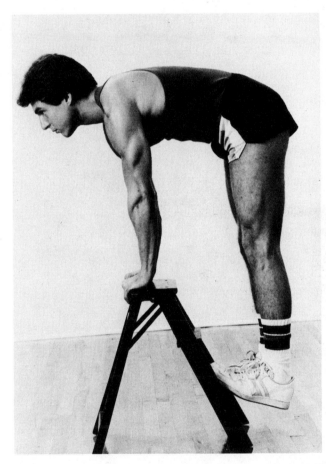

DAYS 2, 4

Basic:	3 sets of 18 repetitions
Improved:	3 sets of 25 repetitions
Advanced:	3 sets of 30 repetitions

7/
ONE-LEGGED HEEL DIPS

DAYS 1, 3

Basic:	4 sets of 10 repetitions
Improved:	4 sets of 20 repetitions
Advanced:	4 sets of 25 repetitions

Same exercise as above but using one leg only at a
time. Alternate legs after each set.

8/
TOE CURLS

Sitting on a bench or chair, place a bath towel under your bare feet. With heels flat, roll your toes upward as high as possible. Then curl toes downward and try to pick up the towel with your toes. Keep heels flat.

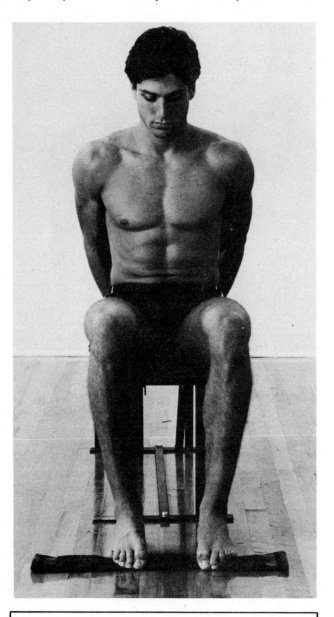 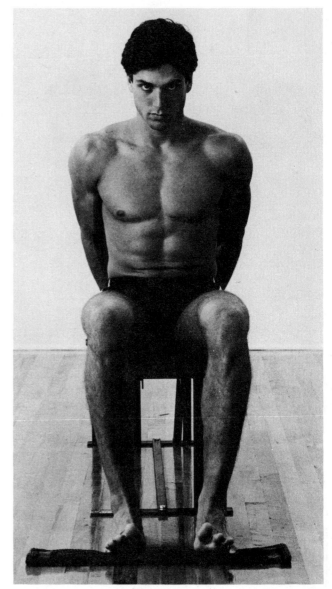

DAYS 2, 4	
Basic:	2 sets of 10 repetitions
Improved:	4 sets of 10 repetitions
Advanced:	4 sets of 15 repetitions

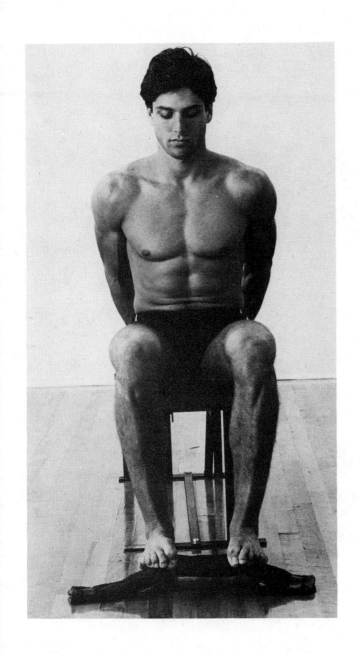

9/
LEG FLUTTERS

Lie flat on a bench face down. Grasp the bench firmly and, keeping legs straight back, flutter your legs as in swimming. You'll be more comfortable with a pad on the bench.

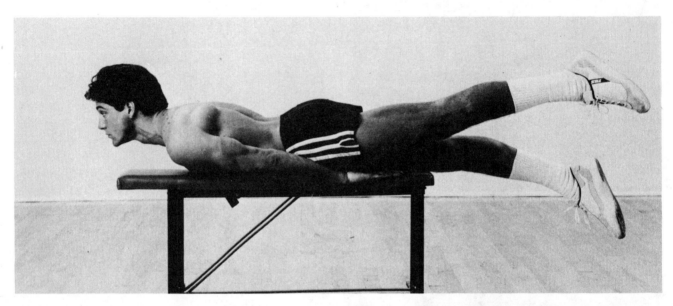

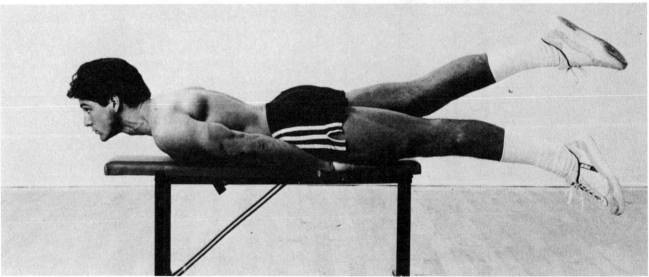

DAYS 1, 3	
Basic:	4 sets of 60 repetitions
Improved:	5 sets of 60 repetitions
Advanced:	6 sets of 60 repetitions

10/
SIDE-TO-SIDE BOUNCE

Place a towel, cushion, or newspaper on the floor alongside your right foot. Starting from a slight crouch, jump sideways over the obstacle and then jump back. Keep to an even rhythm.

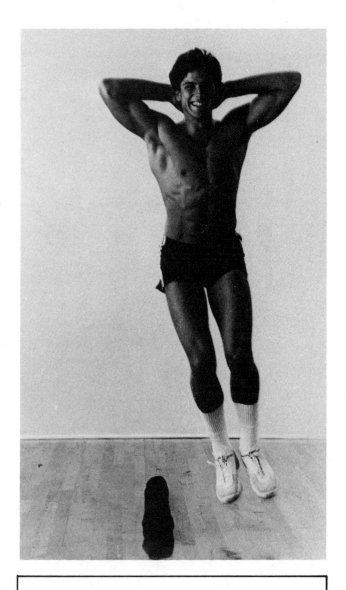 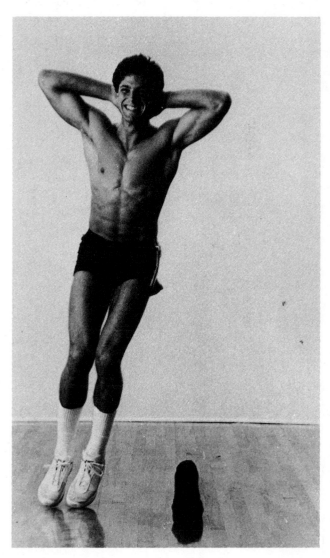

DAYS 2, 4

Basic:	3 sets of 20 repetitions
Improved:	3 sets of 30 repetitions
Advanced:	4 sets of 25 repetitions

11/
SOLEUS TEST AND FLEXION

The soleus is your heel cord. Most sports require you to flex your foot muscles, but few require stretching, which is why you must do it on your own. Test your soleus flexibility by standing with toes two inches from a wall. Keeping heels flat on floor, bend knees until they touch wall. Now move back an inch at a time to see the toe distance at which you keep heels flat and still touch knees. This varies, of course, for leg length, but keep trying to improve the distance from the wall. Exercise: Stand with outstretched arms against wall. Stretch left foot as far back as possible and then right foot forward. Flatten left heel to floor and bend right knee. Keep left foot as far back as possible with heel flat on each bend. Repeat, reversing legs.

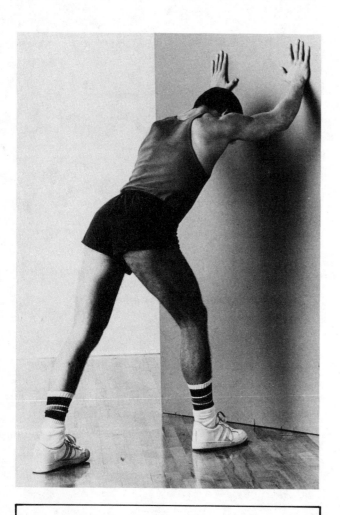

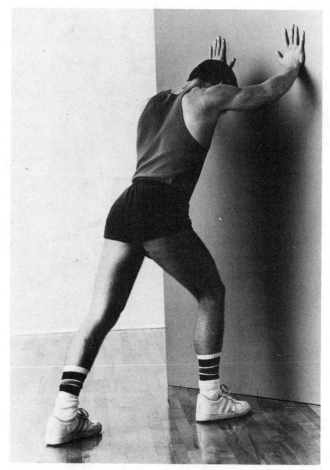

DAYS 1, 3

Basic:	4 sets of 7 repetitions
Improved:	4 sets of 10 repetitions
Advanced:	4 sets of 15 repetitions

12/
CLIMB-UPS

You can start this exercise with an ordinary step and then work up to a foot-high box and finally to a solid chair. The exercise consists in stepping up with one foot on the object and then the other. Then the first foot down, followed by the second. The second set begins with the opposite foot.

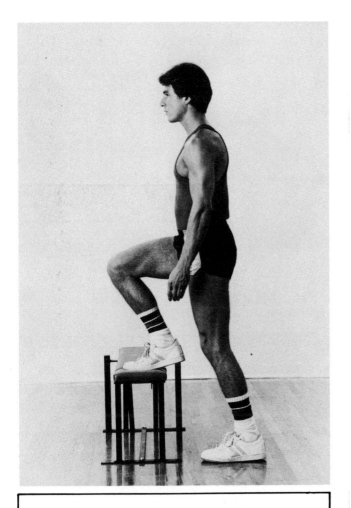

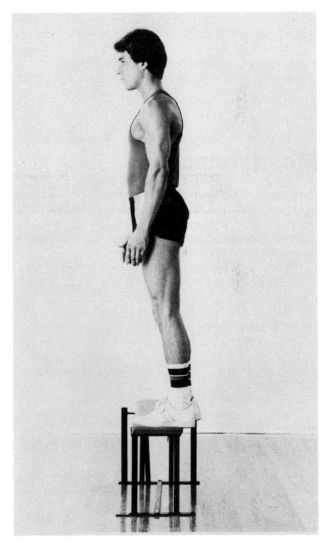

DAYS 2, 4

Basic:	2 sets of 35 repetitions
Improved:	3 sets of 30 repetitions
Advanced:	3 sets of 35 repetitions

Cool-down

Cooling down after a hard workout or game is as important as warming up. Never go straight to the showers. Runners usually jog slowly or walk to cool off. Many athletes raise their arms and "grab sky" as they walk, opening and shutting fists. Follow this with stretching exercises 1, 2, 5, and 6. Remember: Stretching is the best way to cool down. The two important goals to accomplish are to let your heart slow down gradually, and to get all the extra stretching you can while your muscles are warm and limber. If you are thirsty, replace lost body moisture with water or diluted fruit juice. Drinking liquid at this point is good for you.

Maintenance

By the end of the sixth week of accelerating workouts, your body tone should be up to participation in almost any sport at a good level of proficiency. If you're intent on becoming a top competitor, you can skip straight to Chapter VIII.

If you now want to specialize for a particular sport or sports, you can skip to Chapter X. In either case, you should check out Chapter IX to be sure that you're providing the right mix of fuel for the energy you're going to need.

Whichever direction you choose, the most important thing to remember is that fitness is not like ice skating or bridge or driving a car. You can't be away from it for a couple of months or years and then come back and pick up where you left off. Fitness is not like a college degree, which once acquired stays with you the rest of your life. Fitness should be habit-forming; it's one of the few habits in this world that you should never kick.

A maintenance system favored by some trainers is to take a program such as you will have gone through above and, after finishing, take a week off except for stretching and aerobics (which you should never stop) and then start the exercise program over from the beginning. Notice how much easier it becomes the second time around. Notice that you'll be able to handle more sets, more repetitions, with ease. And above all, notice that once you've arrived at this point, the whole program seems to be more fun.

Take a good look at yourself in a full-length mirror. If you like what you see, hang a motto over the mirror. Let it read, "Stay as fit as you are."

CHAPTER V: FITNESS PROGRAM FOR THE COMPETITIVE FEMALE

Women athletes are closing the gap.

That is the almost unanimous opinion of trainers, athletes, and sports medicine experts associated with the Olympic program. Women are approximately 30 years behind men in sports and athletics, but they're moving up in all events except those involving heavy musculature.

The very first participation by women in the Olympics came when demurely costumed ladies entered in figure skating and mixed pairs competition in 1908. In 1912, females were admitted to the summer games but only in swimming events. Fanny Durack of Australia was awarded a gold medal when she swam the 100-meter freestyle in 1:22.2. Then Great Britain's team won the 400-meter freestyle relay in what was regarded as the splendid time of 5:52.8. (The current Olympic record for this event, held by East Germany, is 3:42.71.)

Women were finally allowed to participate in track and field events in 1928, some 32 years after the start of the modern Olympics. They took part in only 5 sports; today, they participate in well over 40 events, including everything from table tennis to judo, with more being added in each successive Olympiad.

Women began to achieve world fame with their Olympic victories when the immortal Sonja Henie of Norway won the figure skating singles in 1928, 1932, and 1936, and turned the sport into an international favorite with her Ice Spectaculars and Hollywood films.

After a long, uphill battle, women athletes are finally being accorded the same respect, attention, and training facilities as men. In large part this is due to the fact that sports medicine authorities and sports physiologists have finally concluded that outside of minor distinctions of body structure and muscle-building capabilities, there are no differences, in athletic terms, between male and female anatomies.

The sensational marathon record that was set by the great Emil Zapotek of Czechoslovakia in 1952 has now been bettered by a woman, and virtually all of today's top women swimmers are beating the times that won gold medals for Don Schollander in the 1964 Olympics.

Trainers are well aware that a woman's heart and lung functions do not differ significantly from a man's, and so there are no longer distinct "female" training routines. Stretching, aerobic, and muscle-building exercises are virtually identical. Weight lifting is usually included in women's body-building routines now that it has been firmly established that hormonal controls do not allow women to develop masculine-type bulging muscles.

The fact that women generally surpass men in flexibility and grace has led women into such distinctive sports as rhythmic gymnastics and synchronous swimming, which require arduous conditioning for lovely and graceful expression.

Turning first to the warm-up, we start with a few of the exercises that women can almost invariably do better than men.

1/
KNEE LIFTS

Stand erect, feet together, arms at sides. Raise your left knee as high as you can clasp it with both hands to your chest. Return to starting position. Repeat with right leg. Alternate legs. 10 repetitions.

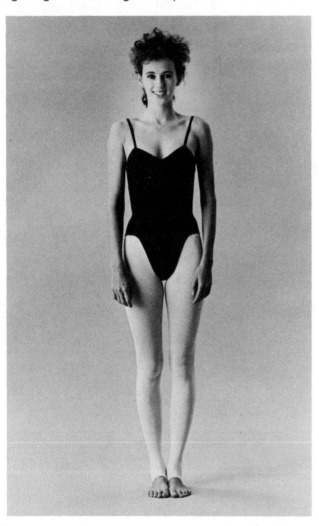 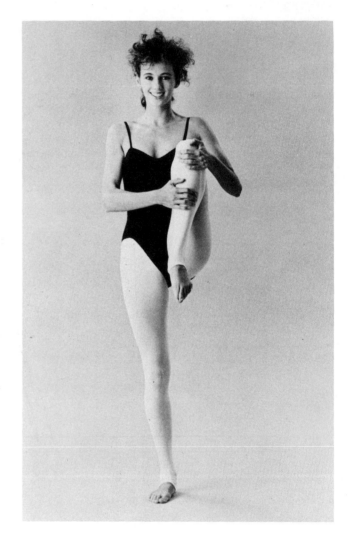

2/
HAMSTRING STRETCH

From a squatting position with hands flat on the
ground and feet slightly apart, straighten your legs,
keeping hands flat on the ground before you. Return.
10 repetitions

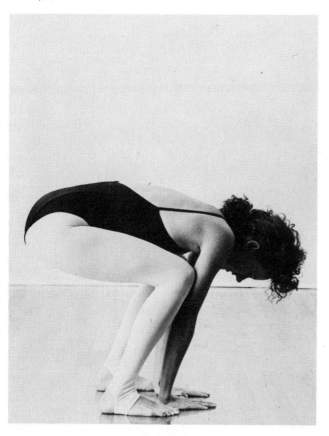 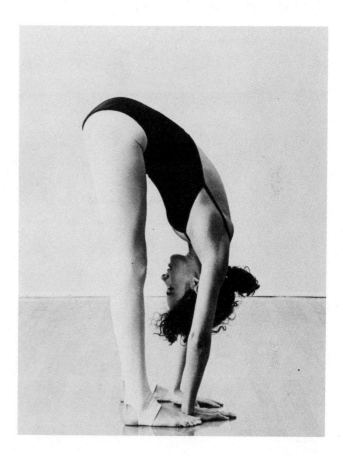

3/
BACK ROLL

Lying flat on your back, knees bent and feet flat down
with arms outstretched above your head, roll your
legs over your head until your toes touch down at
your fingertips. Return. 10 repetitions

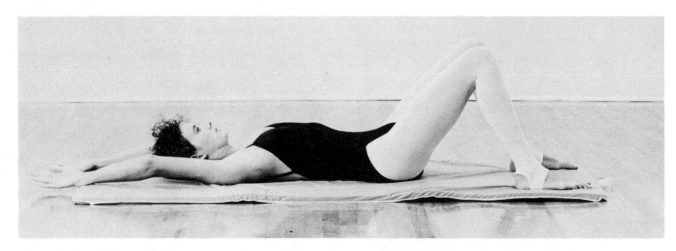

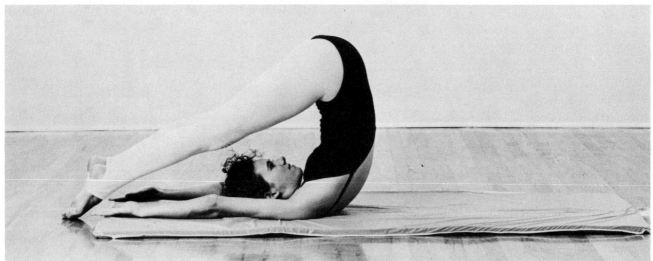

4/
SCISSORS

Lie on your right side with your right arm extended on the floor above your head. Lift your left leg about 2 feet off the floor and lower it. Turn onto your left side with left arm extended and do the same for right leg. 2 sets 10 repetitions each

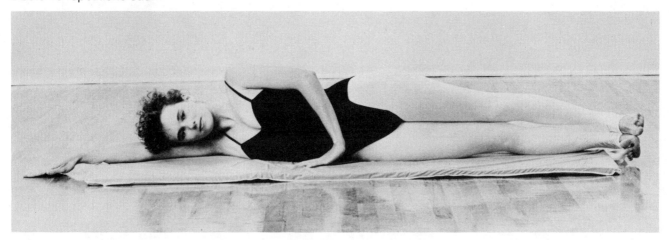

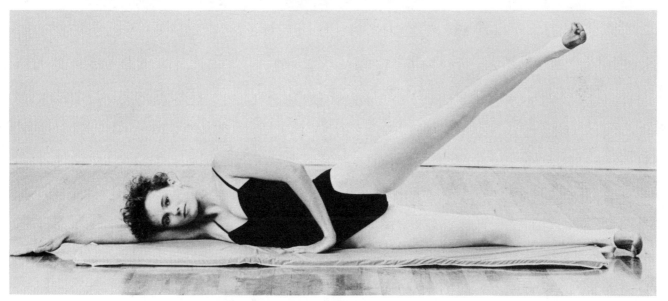

5/
FORWARD ROLL

Lie on your back, legs together, knees bent, and arms stretched above your head. Rise to a sitting position and then slide your hands forward along your legs to your ankles, straightening your knees as you do, and then back all the way. 5 repetitions

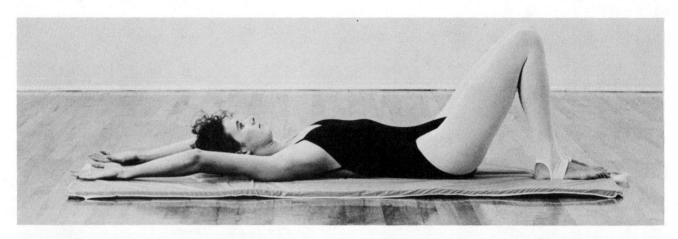

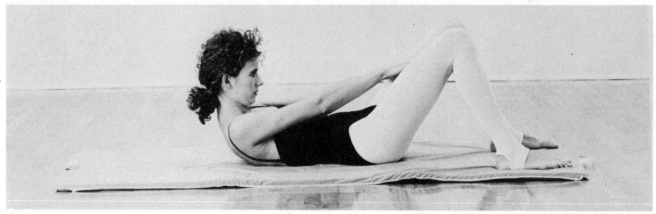

6/
ACHILLES' LIMBER-UP

Stand at arm's length from a wall, feet apart and flat on the floor. Lean against the wall and then bend your elbows until your head touches the wall, keeping your feet flat on the ground. Return after 20 seconds. 4 repetitions

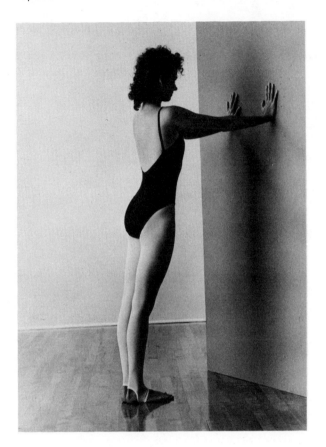
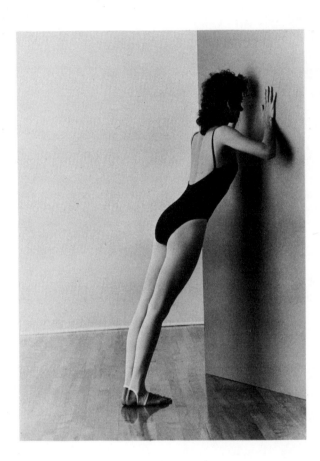

7/
PUSH-UP

Lean against a chair, bend elbows, and do a
straight-body push-up. 5 repetitions

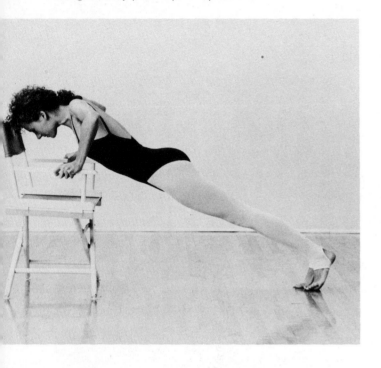 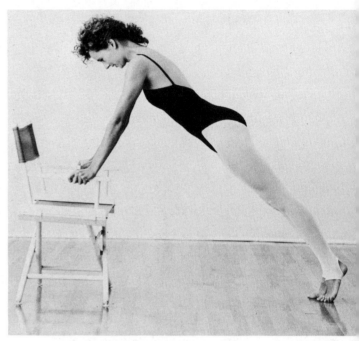

8/
RUN AND JUMPS

Run in place to a count of 60, lifting each foot at least 4 inches off the ground. Then do 10 saddle hops (stand erect, hands at sides, feet together, raise hands straight above your head and clap, jumping legs about 2 feet apart to a straddle position). Do 10 hops and return to start. 2 sets of 60 count running and 10 hops

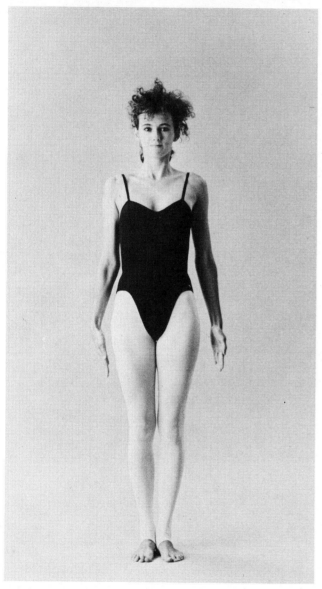
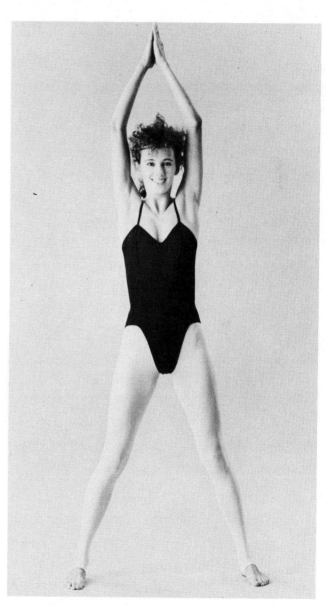

1/
OVER AND UNDER

Start with your arms high above your head, feet apart and hands together. Bend forward and swing your hands between your legs to touch the floor as far be-hind you as you can reach. Straighten up and repeat. 5 repetitions

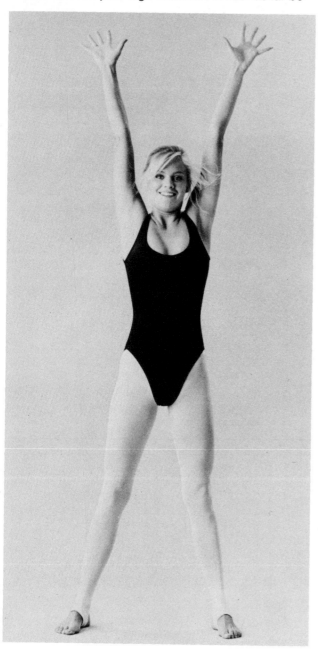

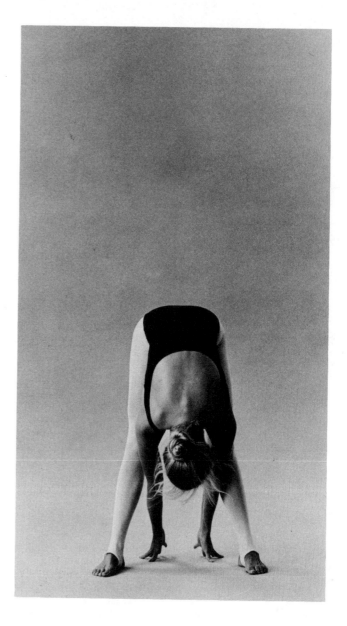

2/
FROG STRETCH

With your feet flat on the floor and legs spread as wide open as you can manage, move your hands to hold your ankles. Raise and lower your hips 4 or 5 times. 2 sets 10 repetitions

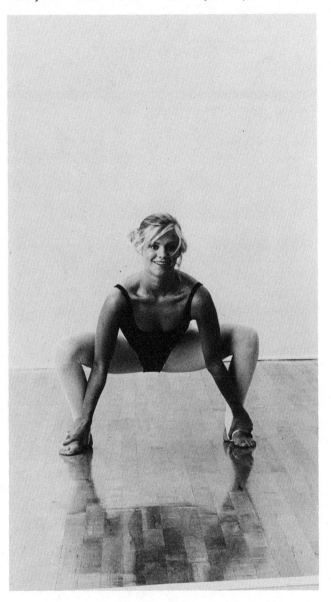
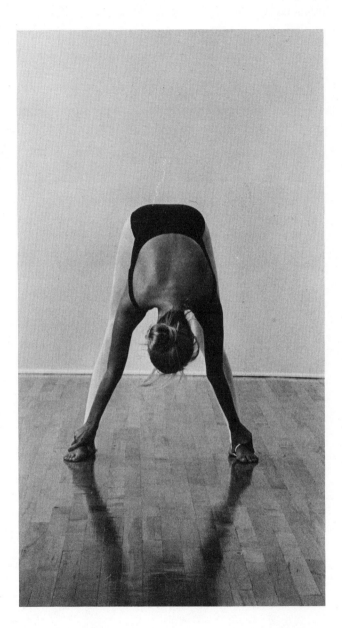

3/
TORSO TWIST

With hands clasped behind your neck, bend forward at the waist until your back is at a right angle to your legs. With elbows straight out, turn until your left el-bow points toward the floor. Slowly twist until your right elbow points toward the floor. Stand erect and repeat. 5 repetitions

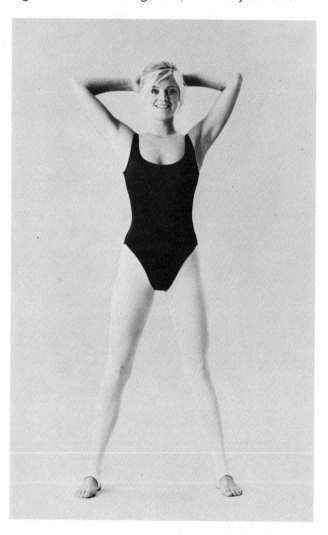 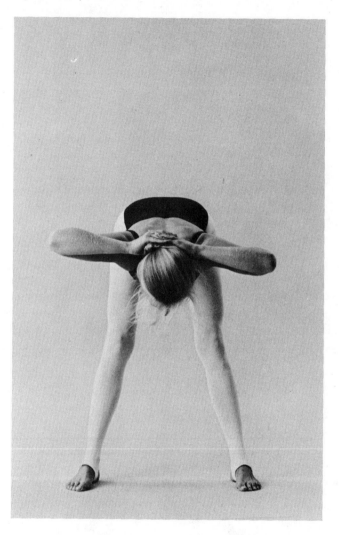

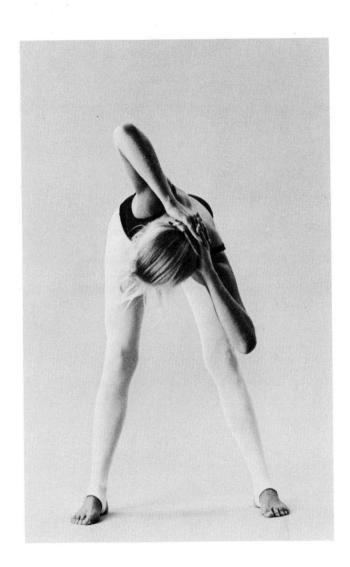

4/
TOE TOUCHES

Stand with your feet apart and arms extended from shoulders. Bending from waist, touch left toe with right hand. Return to erect position. Repeat, touching right toe with left hand (not too fast). 30 seconds

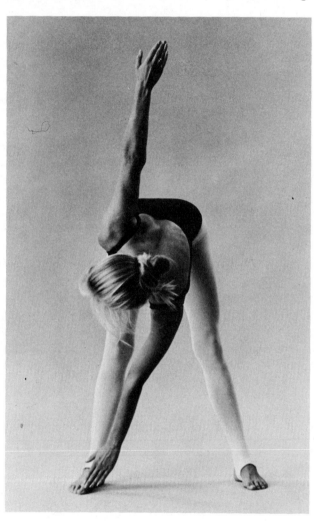 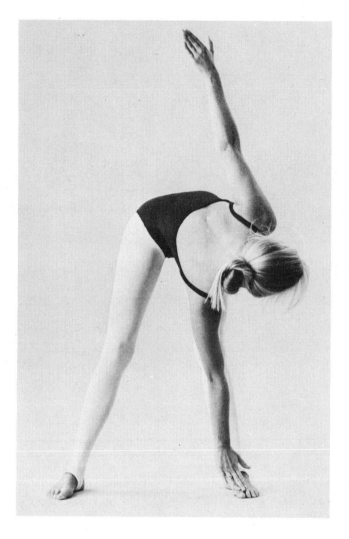

5/
SPINE CURL

Lie on your back with your knees bent and raised,
arms clasped in front of you. Rise to a sitting position,
then bend forward and try to touch chin to knees. Return to supine position. 15 seconds, 3 repetitions

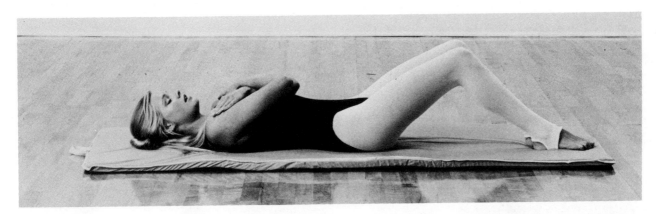

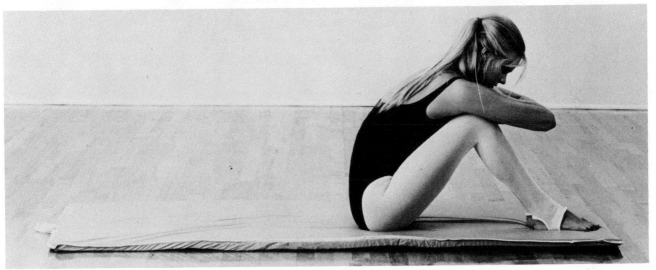

6/
ACHILLES' FLEX

Stand on the edge of a step, your weight on the balls
of your feet. Hold wall or bannister for balance. Dip
your heels down as far as you can go. 15 seconds, 3
repetitions

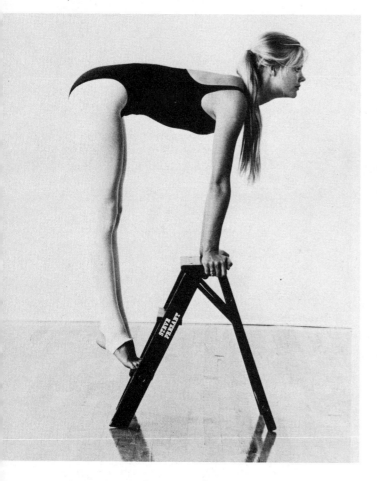
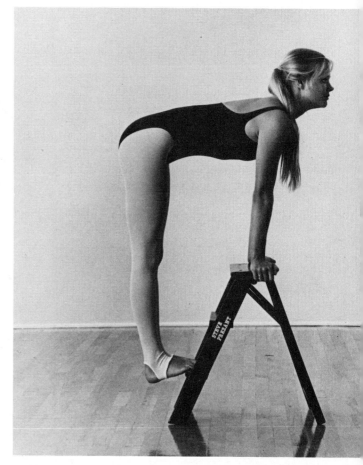

Aerobic Conditioning

Refer back to the section on aerobic conditioning for the male athlete (page 57).

You may make a gender allowance of up to 10 percent on the running, cycling, and swimming minimums, but women are well able to keep up with men in aerobic sports, as anyone who has ever witnessed a marathon can attest. You may substitute aerobic disco dancing for running in place or rope skipping so long as you continue steadily for at least 20 minutes.

You may also decide to choose one of the following aerobic exercises:

1. Running or jogging—1 mile in 12 minutes or less
2. Swimming—30 laps in 30 minutes or less in a 60-foot pool
3. Cycling—3 miles in 15 minutes (twice daily if possible); you may follow the same schedule on a stationary bicycle
4. Walking—1 mile in 25 minutes (four times daily if possible)
5. Aerobic dancing, rhythmic gymnastics, or rope skipping— vigorous 20 minutes (you may take 4 1-minute rest periods if you need them)

The above schedule is for top aerobic endurance. For sports requiring lesser cardiovascular and respiratory capability, the above aerobics may be scaled down. But remember that it is always better to exceed your requirement than to undercondition yourself.

Exercises for the Competitive Female

The 32 exercises that follow, divided into the three main body areas, are identical to the exercises given for male athletes in Chapter IV—the sets and repetitions have been slightly modified. Refer back to pages 60—95 for descriptions and photographs.

The exercise schedule is based on four sessions a week, though it can be reduced to three if time or facilities are limited. Do odd-numbered exercises on days 1 and 3 of your four-day exercise schedule and do even-numbered exercises on days 2 and 4. If you cannot do all of the repetitions, do as many as you can and go on to the next exercise, staying in sequence. When you have finished the routine, rest for a short period, drink water or diluted fruit juice if you're thirsty, and then go back and try to finish the uncompleted exercises. If you miss an exercise schedule, try to perform the stretching exercises and some aerobic activity. So far as possible, stretching out and aerobics should be part of your daily lifestyle.

No part of a woman's body is at more of a disadvantage to a man's muscular strength than the forearms. Therefore, any exercise that involves push-ups can be done pushing up from a chair rather than the floor. Likewise, the woman's modified chin-up allows you to stand on a box or low platform, take the chin-up position, and then lower yourself to a straight hangdown. Repetitions are done by climbing back on the box each time to start the exercise.

1/
Push-ups   *(See page 60.)*

Push up from bent knees or from a chair if necessary.

DAYS 1, 3	
Basic:	2 sets of 6 repetitions
Improved:	3 sets of 6 repetitions
Advanced:	4 sets of 5 repetitions

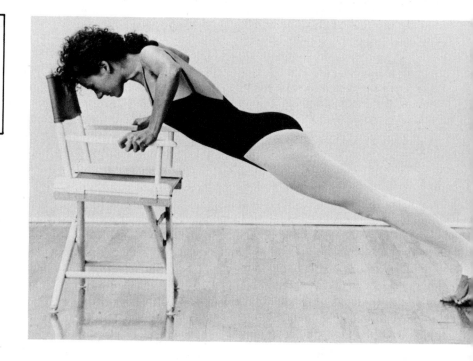

2/
Pump-ups   *(See page 61.)*

DAYS 2, 4	
Basic:	2 sets of 4 repetitions
Improved:	3 sets of 5 repetitions
Advanced:	3 sets of 6 repetitions

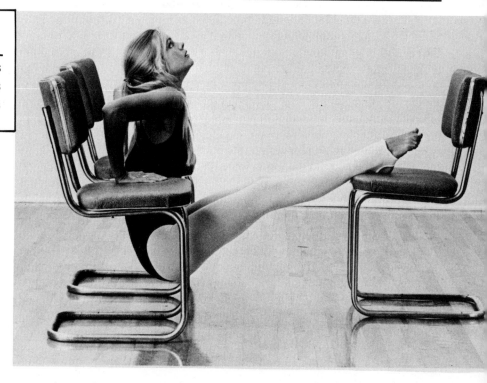

3/
Chin-ups *(See page 62.)*

If you cannot pull yourself up, stand on a box, grasp
the bar, and slowly ease yourself down.

DAYS 1, 3	
Basic:	1 set of 7 repetitions
Improved:	2 sets of 5 repetitions
Advanced:	2 sets of 5 repetitions

4/
French Curl *(See page 63.)*

You may use dumbbells instead of the barbell.

DAYS 2, 4	
Basic:	2 sets of 5 repetitions
Improved:	3 sets of 4 repetitions
Advanced:	3 sets of 5 repetitions

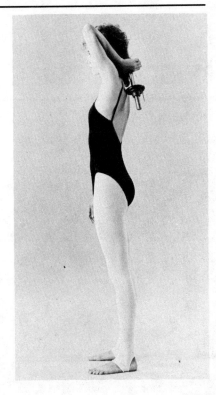

5/
Wrist Curl   *(See page 64.)*

You may use dumbbells instead of the barbell.

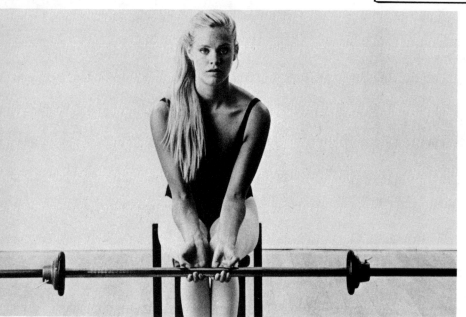

6/
Bench Press   *(See page 65.)*

You may use dumbbells instead of the barbell.

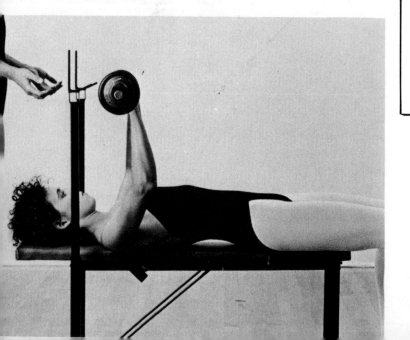

7/
Biceps Curl *(See page 66.)*

You may use dumbbells instead of the barbell.

DAYS 1, 3		
Basic:	3 sets of 6 repetitions
Improved:	3 sets of 7 repetitions
Advanced:	3 sets of 8 repetitions

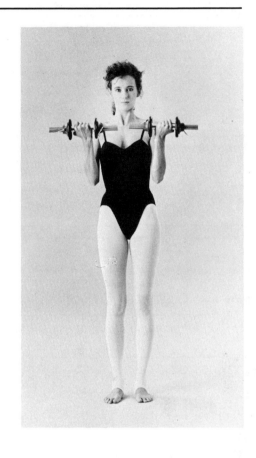

8/
Butterfly Swing *(See page 67.)*

DAYS 2, 4		
Basic:	3 sets of 4 repetitions
Improved:	2 sets of 7 repetitions
Advanced:	2 sets of 7 repetitions

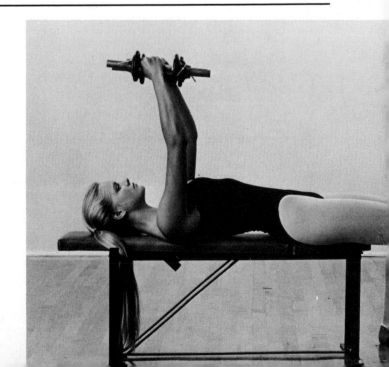

9/
Ball Clutch *(See page 68.)*

DAYS 1, 3	
Basic:	2 sets of 8 repetitions
Improved:	5 sets of 8 repetitions
Advanced:	7 sets of 8 repetitions

10/
Towel Wring *(See page 68.)*

DAYS 2, 4	
Basic:	2 sets of 4 repetitions
Improved:	3 sets of 5 repetitions
Advanced:	4 sets of 6 repetitions

The Mid Body

1/
Bent-knee Sit-ups *(See page 69.)*

DAYS 1, 3	
Basic:	2 sets of 6 repetitions
Improved:	3 sets of 6 repetitions
Advanced:	3 sets of 8 repetitions

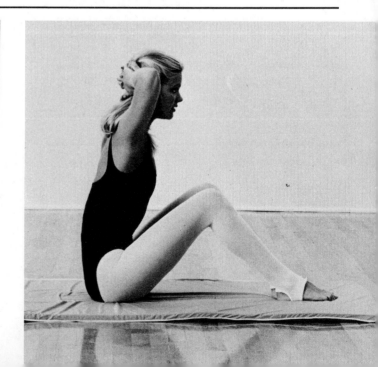

2/
Leg Lifts *(See page 70.)*

DAYS 2, 4	
Basic:	1 set of 15 repetitions
Improved:	2 sets of 10 repetitions
Advanced:	2 sets of 12 repetitions

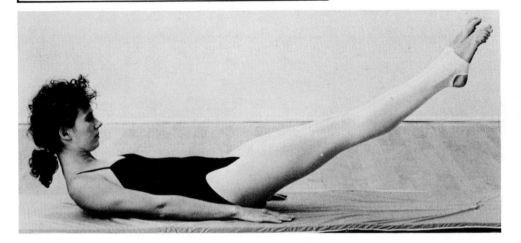

3/
Dumbbell Lifts *(See page 71.)*

DAYS 1, 3	
Basic:	2 sets of 15 repetitions
Improved:	3 sets of 12 repetitions
Advanced:	3 sets of 12 repetitions

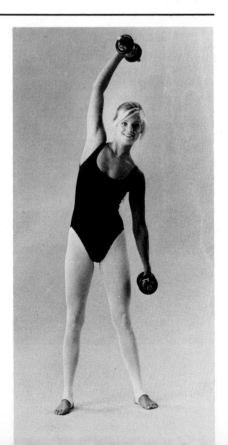

4/
Foot Lifts *(See page 72.)*

DAYS 2, 4	
Basic:	1 set of 20 repetitions
Improved:	2 sets of 12 repetitions
Advanced:	3 sets of 9 repetitions

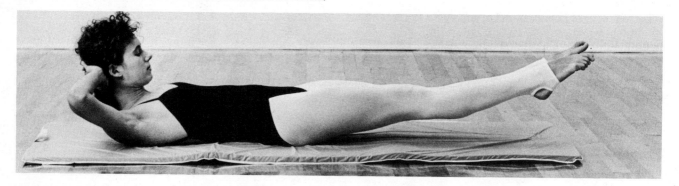

5/
Lift-offs *(See page 73.)*

DAYS 1, 3	
Basic:	3 sets of 8 repetitions
Improved:	3 sets of 12 repetitions
Advanced:	3 sets of 12 repetitions

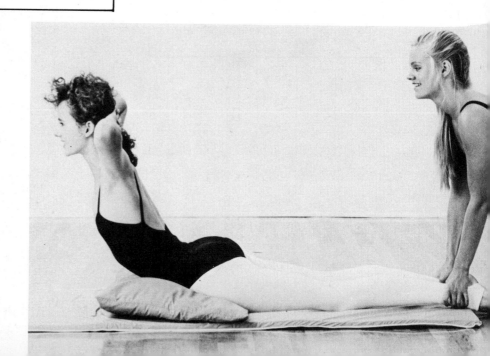

6/
Round-up Twist *(See page 74.)*

(See page 74.)

DAYS 2, 4	
Basic:	2 sets of 12 repetitions
Improved:	3 sets of 9 repetitions
Advanced:	3 sets of 10 repetitions

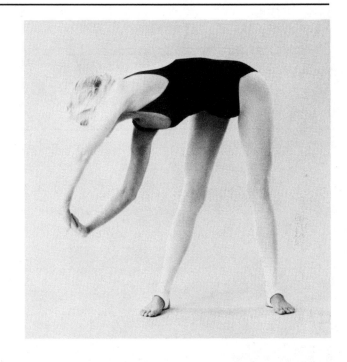

7/
Torso Torsion *(See page 76.)*

(See page 76.)

DAYS 1, 3	
Basic:	2 sets of 5 repetitions
Improved:	3 sets of 5 repetitions
Advanced:	3 sets of 10 repetitions

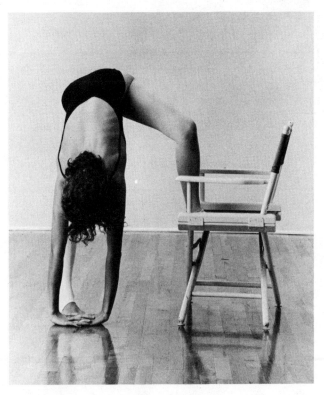

8/
Punting Practice *(See page 78.)*

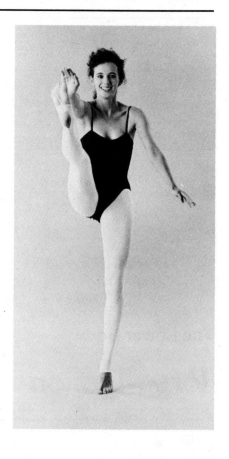

DAYS 2, 4	
Basic:	2 sets of 5 repetitions
Improved:	2 sets of 10 repetitions
Advanced:	3 sets of 8 repetitions

9/
Weight Swing *(See page 80.)*

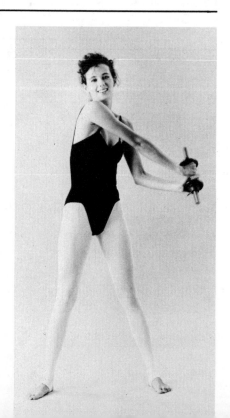

DAYS 1, 3	
Basic:	3 sets of 12 repetitions
Improved:	3 sets of 12 repetitions
Advanced:	3 sets of 12 repetitions

10/
Towel Pull *(See page 82.)*

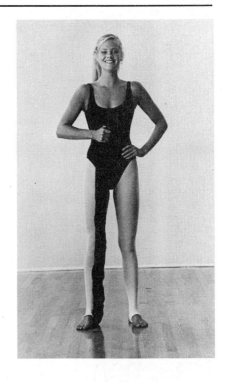

DAYS 2, 4

Basic:	2 sets of 10 repetitions
Improved:	3 sets of 8 repetitions
Advanced:	3 sets of 10 repetitions

The Lower Body

1/
No-chair Sit *(See page 83.)*

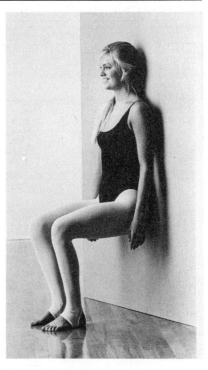

DAYS 1, 3

Basic:	3 sets of 12 repetitions
Improved:	3 sets of 12 repetitions
Advanced:	3 sets of 12 repetitions

2/
Hop-ups *(See page 84.)*

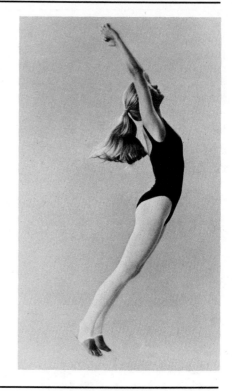

DAYS 2, 4

Basic:	2 sets of 22 repetitions	
Improved:	3 sets of 16 repetitions	
Advanced:	3 sets of 18 repetitions	

3/
Kneebends *(See page 86.)*

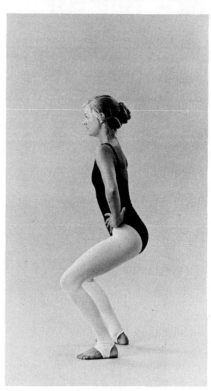

DAYS 1, 3

Basic:	2 sets of 20 repetitions	
Improved:	3 sets of 18 repetitions	
Advanced:	3 sets of 20 repetitions	

4/
Weighted Kneebends *(See page 87.)*

Use dumbbells held above the shoulders until instructor approves use of the barbell.

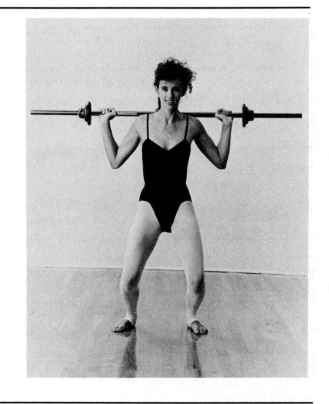

DAYS 2, 4	
Basic:	3 sets of 12 repetitions
Improved:	3 sets of 12 repetitions
Advanced:	3 sets of 15 repetitions

5/
Foot Lifts *(See page 88.)*

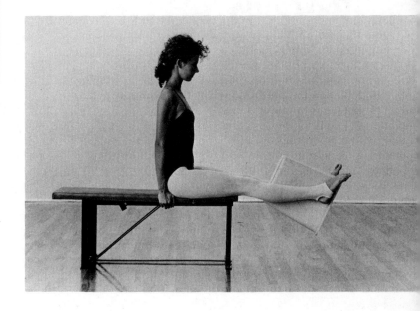

DAYS 1, 3	
Basic:	3 sets of 10 repetitions
Improved:	3 sets of 12 repetitions
Advanced:	3 sets of 12 repetitions

6/
Heel Dips *(See page 89.)*

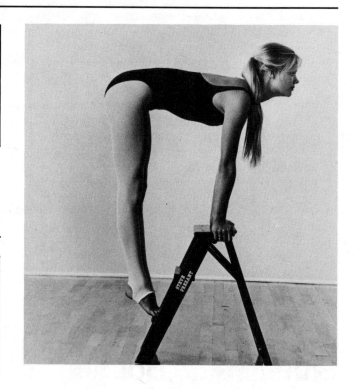

DAYS 2, 4

Basic:	3 sets of 12 repetitions
Improved:	3 sets of 15 repetitions
Advanced:	3 sets of 15 repetitions

7/ *(See page 98.)*
One-legged Heel Dips

DAYS 1, 3

Basic:	3 sets of 8 repetitions
Improved:	4 sets of 10 repetitions
Advanced:	4 sets of 12 repetitions

8/
Toe Curls *(See page 90.)*

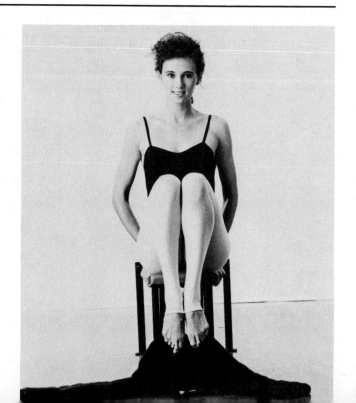

DAYS 2, 4

Basic:	2 sets of 5 repetitions
Improved:	3 sets of 5 repetitions
Advanced:	4 sets of 8 repetitions

9/
Leg Flutters *(See page 92.)*

(See page 92.)

DAYS 1, 3	
Basic:	2 sets of 6 repetitions
Improved:	2 sets of 8 repetitions
Advanced:	2 sets of 10 repetitions

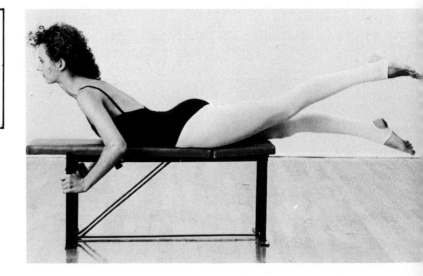

10/
Side-to-side Bounce *(See page 93.)*

(See page 93.)

Use a book to jump over to start.

DAYS 2, 4	
Basic:	3 sets of 7 repetitions
Improved:	3 sets of 9 repetitions
Advanced:	3 sets of 10 repetitions

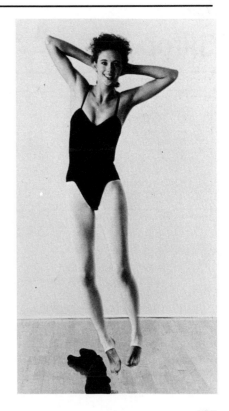

11/
Soleus Test and Flexion *(See page 94.)*

(See page 94.)

DAYS 1, 3

Basic:	2 sets of 10 repetitions
Improved:	3 sets of 10 repetitions
Advanced:	4 sets of 10 repetitions

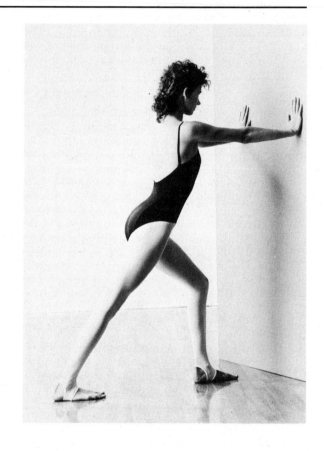

12/
Climb-ups *(See page 95.)*

(See page 95.)

DAYS 2, 4

Basic:	2 sets of 18 repetitions
Improved:	3 sets of 18 repetitions
Advanced:	3 sets of 20 repetitions

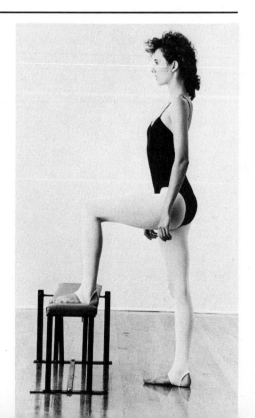

Cool-down

Follow same routine as that given in Chapter IV for male athletes.

Maintenance

Women are closing the athletic gap with men in many sports, but our society still maintains many sexual stereotypes. As a female athlete, you may find yourself shunted again and again into sedentary jobs; because of this and related factors, it is always an uphill battle for a woman to keep athletically fit. But it can be done. More and more women are doing it—and enjoying it—and living happier, more healthy lives for it.

But the big point to remember is this: Fitness is not a sometimes thing. Fitness is an always thing.

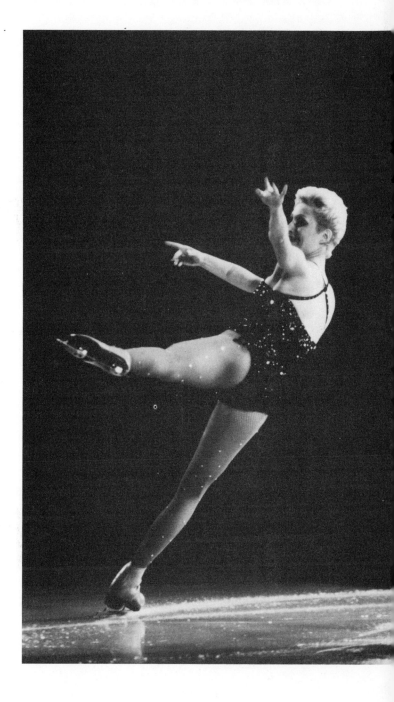

I like to win. And I guess I've got some kind of drive that others don't. At this level, where we're almost all in the same physical condition, that's what sets the winners apart.
—Tracy Caulkins, The Olympian, June/July 1979

CHAPTER VI: FITNESS PROGRAM FOR THE ATHLETIC ADOLESCENT MALE

At what age should a boy start training to be an athlete? American Olympic coaches and trainers are unanimous in rejecting the Soviet system of starting kids in a rigorous training routine at 5 or 6.
They feel that at this age, boys should come to sports in the form of games and neighborhood play. Basketball, baseball, football, volley ball, ice and field hockey, and similar running and throwing games are great for the youngster of 8 and 10.

Bob Beeten, associate director of sports medicine for the U.S. Olympic Training Center in Colorado Springs, feels that if a boy gets too seriously involved in sports at too early an age, he stops having fun as he grows older, and competition becomes a grind. Beeten points out that as kids change, their interests change. Often the sport they're first attracted to isn't the sport they want to play as they grow more mature. Most of the real sports interest, he says, begins to develop at 14 or 15 and goes on through the growth period.

John Anderson, basketball trainer at Louisiana State and trainer of Olympic aspirants at the Olympic Training Center, feels that a basketball player should be into the sport by 10 and learn team play and competition in high school. Jim Fox, director of the Amateur Boxing Federation, thinks 10 is a good age for a boy to learn to use the gloves. If the boy is serious, he says, the first requirement is to get with a good coach and learn the fundamentals; then get into a state group-development program. Gordie Genz, volley ball coach at Purdue University and trainer of Olympic talent, also feels that 8 to 10 is a good age for a boy to get into that sport. "Great basketball players are born," he maintains, "but great volley ball players are made."

For games like soccer and field hockey, Alex Stanopovich, team manager of field hockey at the National Sports Festival, feels "you can't begin too young" but qualifies that to mean around 8 for serious neighborhood game play.

Bob Beeten reminds us that girls develop earlier than boys and have gone through the major portion of their growth cycle by 13 or 14, whereas for boys it's about two years later. Only after that point has been passed, he suggests, should serious aerobic and weight training begin. As the youthful athlete gets into competition, he can work out as many as five to seven times a week. However, an hour and a half per session is about the maximum period for which a young athlete can maintain the required intensity and concentration.

The physical fitness of American youngsters has been a matter of deep concern to the American gov-

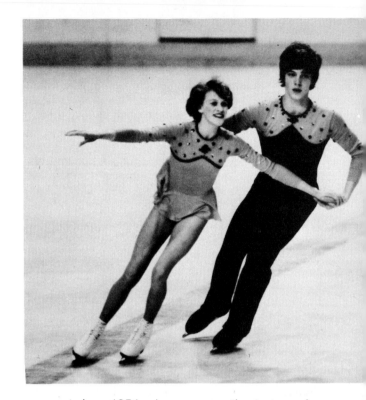

ernment since 1954, when comparative tests on Austrian, Italian, Swiss, and American children showed a failure rate almost five times as high among the U.S. youth in meeting minimum fitness standards.
The direct consequence of this was the creation of The President's Council on Physical Fitness; the ultimate consequence was that in the course of thirty years, Americans finally became fitness oriented and are now in the process of catching up with the rest of the world.

The following exercise routines are directed toward young men who have passed puberty, are at least 15 or 16 years of age, and are serious about competitive athletics.

Warm-up

As an adolescent athlete, you will have no trouble following the warm-up program outlined in Chapter IV, page 57. Your youthful muscles will be slimmer but more supple than those of your seniors. We offer this counsel, however: If you come into this program without any previous training beyond casual school gym classes, you can start with about two-thirds the number of repetitions and work your way up to the indicated quota.

Stretching

Mastery of the stretching exercises is extremely important. If you can resolve to keep yourself physically fit for the rest of your life, you'll still be doing these or similar stretching routines as a senior citizen. Don't be tempted to rush into the body of the exercise routines without at least 20 minutes to a half hour of warm-up and stretching.

Aerobic Conditioning

If you haven't had previous running training, physiologists recommend starting the aerobics program on an every-other-day basis. Muscle growth is directly proportional to the intensity of the exercise. To keep up a high intensity as the muscles develop, you should give them 48 hours of rest between workouts. However, it doesn't follow that if a day's rest is good, two days' rest is better. It isn't. You've got to keep at it. At age 13, you should be able to cover 1½ miles in about 11 minutes. At 19, you should have this time down to 9½ minutes or better. The same ratio goes for the swimming, biking, walking, or rope-skipping equivalents of running.

Exercises for the Adolescent Male

The 32 exercises that follow, divided into the three main body areas, are identical to the exercises given in Chapter IV—the sets and repetitions have been slightly modified. Refer back to pages 60—95 for descriptions and photographs.

The exercise schedule is based on four sessions a week, though it can be reduced to three if time or facilities are limited. Do odd-numbered exercises on days 1 and 3 of your four-day exercise schedule and do even-numbered exercises on days 2 and 4. If you cannot do all of the repetitions, do as many as you can and go on to the next exercise, staying in sequence. When you have finished the routine, rest for a short period, drink water or diluted fruit juice if you're thirsty, and then go back and try to finish the uncompleted exercises. If you miss an exercise schedule, try to perform the stretching exercises and some aerobic activity. So far as possible, stretching and aerobics should be part of your daily lifestyle.

But you're not really a machine. There is life after skating.
—Scott Hamilton, 1983 U.S. figure skating champion

1/
Push-ups *(See page 60.)*

You may push up from a chair if you wish.

```
DAYS 1, 3
───────────────────────────────────
        Basic:    3 sets of 10 repetitions
     Improved:    4 sets of 10 repetitions
     Advanced:    4 sets of 12 repetitions
```

2/
Pump-ups *(See page 61.)*

```
DAYS 2, 4
───────────────────────────────────
        Basic:    2 sets of 7 repetitions
     Improved:    2 sets of 12 repetitions
     Advanced:    2 sets of 15 repetitions
```

3/
Chin-ups *(See page 62.)*

If you cannot pull yourself up, stand on a box, grasp the bar, and slowly ease yourself down.

```
DAYS 1, 3
───────────────────────────────────
        Basic:    3 sets of 7 repetitions
     Improved:    3 sets of 10 repetitions
     Advanced:    3 sets of 12 repetitions
```

4/
French Curl *(See page 63.)*

You may use dumbbells instead of the barbell.

DAYS 2, 4

Basic:	2 sets of 12 repetitions
Improved:	3 sets of 10 repetitions
Advanced:	3 sets of 12 repetitions

5/
Wrist Curl *(See page 64.)*

You may use dumbbells instead of the barbell.

DAYS 1, 3

Basic:	3 sets of 8 repetitions
Improved:	3 sets of 12 repetitions
Advanced:	3 sets of 15 repetitions

6/
Bench Press *(See page 65.)*

You may use dumbbells instead of the barbell.

DAYS 2, 4

Basic:	3 sets of 10 repetitions
Improved:	3 sets of 12 repetitions
Advanced:	3 sets of 15 repetitions

7/
Biceps Curl   *(See page 66.)*

You may use dumbbells instead of the barbell.

DAYS 1, 3	
Basic:	4 sets of 5 repetitions
Improved:	2 sets of 10 repetitions
Advanced:	2 sets of 12 repetitions

8/
Butterfly Swing   *(See page 67.)*

DAYS 2, 4	
Basic:	3 sets of 5 repetitions
Improved:	2 sets of 9 repetitions
Advanced:	2 sets of 10 repetitions

9/
Ball Clutch   *(See page 68.)*

DAYS 1, 3	
Basic:	4 sets of 8 repetitions
Improved:	6 sets of 8 repetitions
Advanced:	8 sets of 12 repetitions

10/
Towel Wring *(See page 68.)*

DAYS 2, 4

Basic:	2 sets of 4 repetitions
Improved:	4 sets of 6 repetitions
Advanced:	5 sets of 6 repetitions

The Mid Body

1/
Bent-knee Sit-ups *(See page 69.)*

DAYS 1, 3

Basic:	2 sets of 12 repetitions
Improved:	3 sets of 12 repetitions
Advanced:	3 sets of 12 repetitions

2/
Leg Lifts *(See page 70.)*

DAYS 2, 4

Basic:	1 set of 18 repetitions
Improved:	2 sets of 12 repetitions
Advanced:	2 sets of 15 repetitions

3/
Dumbbell Lifts   *(See page 71.)*

DAYS 1, 3

Basic:	2 sets of 15 repetitions
Improved:	3 sets of 15 repetitions
Advanced:	3 sets of 15 repetitions

4/
Foot Lifts   *(See page 72.)*

DAYS 2, 4

Basic:	1 set of 25 repetitions
Improved:	2 sets of 15 repetitions
Advanced:	2 sets of 15 repetitions

5/
Lift-offs   *(See page 73.)*

DAYS 1, 3

Basic:	2 sets of 18 repetitions
Improved:	2 sets of 20 repetitions
Advanced:	3 sets of 15 repetitions

6/
Round-up Twist *(See page 74.)*

DAYS 2, 4

Basic:	2 sets of 15 repetitions
Improved:	3 sets of 12 repetitions
Advanced:	3 sets of 12 repetitions

7/
Torso Torsion *(See page 76.)*

DAYS 1, 3

Basic:	2 sets of 8 repetitions
Improved:	3 sets of 8 repetitions
Advanced:	3 sets of 10 repetitions

8/
Punting Practice *(See page 78.)*

DAYS 2, 4

Basic:	2 sets of 5 repetitions
Improved:	3 sets of 8 repetitions
Advanced:	3 sets of 10 repetitions

9/
Weight Swing *(See page 80.)*

DAYS 1, 3

Basic:	3 sets of 12 repetitions
Improved:	3 sets of 15 repetitions
Advanced:	3 sets of 15 repetitions

10/
Towel Pull *(See page 82.)*

DAYS 2, 4

Basic:	2 sets of 12 repetitions
Improved:	2 sets of 15 repetitions
Advanced:	2 sets of 15 repetitions

The Lower Body

1/
No-chair Sit *(See page 83.)*

DAYS 1, 3

Basic:	3 sets of 18 repetitions
Improved:	3 sets of 20 repetitions
Advanced:	3 sets of 20 repetitions

2/
Hop-ups *(See page 84.)*

DAYS 2, 4

Basic:	2 sets of 30 repetitions
Improved:	3 sets of 25 repetitions
Advanced:	3 sets of 25 repetitions

3/
Kneebends *(See page 86.)*

DAYS 1, 3

Basic:	2 sets of 25 repetitions
Improved:	3 sets of 20 repetitions
Advanced:	3 sets of 25 repetitions

4/
Weighted Kneebends *(See page 87.)*

You may use dumbbells instead of the barbell.

DAYS 2, 4

Basic:	3 sets of 12 repetitions
Improved:	3 sets of 18 repetitions
Advanced:	3 sets of 20 repetitions

5/
Foot Lifts *(See page 88.)*

DAYS 1, 3

Basic:	3 sets of 12 repetitions
Improved:	3 sets of 15 repetitions
Advanced:	3 sets of 17 repetitions

6/
Heel Dips *(See page 89.)*

DAYS 2, 4

Basic:	3 sets of 17 repetitions
Improved:	3 sets of 20 repetitions
Advanced:	3 sets of 20 repetitions

7/
One-legged Heel Dips *(See page 89.)*

DAYS 1, 3

Basic:	4 sets of 12 repetitions
Improved:	4 sets of 15 repetitions
Advanced:	4 sets of 15 repetitions

8/
Leg Flutters *(See page 92.)*

DAYS 2, 4

Basic:	2 sets of 50 repetitions
Improved:	3 sets of 50 repetitions
Advanced:	4 sets of 50 repetitions

9/
Toe Curls *(See page 90.)*

DAYS 1, 3

Basic:	2 sets of 5 repetitions
Improved:	3 sets of 10 repetitions
Advanced:	4 sets of 10 repetitions

10/
Side-to-side Bounce *(See page 93.)*

DAYS 2, 4

Basic:	4 sets of 7 repetitions
Improved:	4 sets of 8 repetitions
Advanced:	4 sets of 8 repetitions

11/
Soleus Test and Flexion (See page 94.)

(See page 94.)

DAYS 1, 3

Basic:	4 sets of 5 repetitions
Improved:	4 sets of 8 repetitions
Advanced:	4 sets of 10 repetitions

12/
Climb-ups (See page 95.)

(See page 95.)

DAYS 2, 4

Basic:	2 sets of 30 repetitions
Improved:	3 sets of 25 repetitions
Advanced:	3 sets of 25 repetitions

Cool-down

Follow same routine as that given in Chapter IV.

Maintenance

The end result of some three months of strenuous training for the adolescent male athlete is not merely to tone up your body for vigorous participation in the sport of your choice but to give you the kind of physical control over your body that allows you to carry yourself with poise and confidence in your daily life. The teens are inevitably years of insecurity and self-doubt. Athletic competence won't cure that, but it helps—ask any boy.

Twelve weeks of fitness workouts won't make a sports hero out of you. From here on, you need to play your game or practice for your event. You also have to drill in it over and over, week after week after week. Special exercises suited to your sport, as outlined in Chapter X, will help you to compete, but there are no shortcuts in training. The winning edge is achieved, literally, by the sweat of your brow.

If you decide to change sports because you think you'd be better at something else, now's the time to change, before you get locked in. Don't switch simply because you or your team didn't win the championship. One of the hardest lessons that young players have to learn is that "you can't win 'em all." Loss of a hard-fought game or defeat in any sport can sometimes represent so great a sense of personal failure that youngsters need all the support that coaches and parents can give to assure them that there can be life after defeat. Young athletes take their sports very seriously. Families and friends should recognize the magnitude of the disaster they often feel in losing. A smart loser can often get more out of a game than a smug winner.

CHAPTER VII: FITNESS PROGRAM FOR THE ATHLETIC ADOLESCENT FEMALE

A whole new horizon of athletic activity has opened to girls and young women in the past decade. Like an endearing young elf, Nadia Comaneci of Rumania turned gymnastics from a boring exercise routine into a dazzling display of grace and skill in 1976. Gymnastics proved so attractive and so suited to young girls that at the last National Sports Festival, the average age of several of the girls' teams was 14!

Since it's a fact of life that girls usually reach puberty a year or two ahead of boys, strenuous training for girls in such sports as figure skating, swimming, diving, and of course both rhythmic and athletic gymnastics can begin at 13 or 14. Skiing and tennis are not far behind.

The comparatively new sport of rhythmic gymnastics, included in the official Olympic competition for the first time in 1984, is attracting many young women and girls. The grace and agility of the contestant are emphasized by the use of a hoop, a ball, ribbon on a baton, and two skittles, or Indian clubs. The performance, to musical accompaniment, is a thoroughly delightful combination of rhythm, coordination, and athletic elegance.

Synchronous swimming is another fascinating and rewarding event in Olympic competition. As a background, a girl should be a good dancer, preferably in ballet, a good gymnast, and a good swimmer. She needs to have "light" muscular development as opposed to "heavy" muscles; this means that she tends to float rather than sink in the water. Physically, an important element is flexibility; mentally, Olympic coaches require a willing attitude and true dedication.

For the short, slim girl who seriously wants to take part in competitive athletics, Sue Pringle, of the national governing body of the U.S. Field Hockey Association, points out that field hockey offers ideal opportunities. Many top players, including Olympic contestants, are 5 feet 3 inches and even shorter. Gwen Cheeseman, for example, with an all-world ranking, is only 5 feet 2 inches tall. Agility, endurance, and skill in handling the stick are of prime importance.

Figure skating is another extremely attractive area of participation for a girl. Larry McCallum, executive director of the U.S. Figure Skating Association, explains that youngsters are getting better and better in this sport beause they are spending more time in the arena and getting technically proficient at a much earlier age. In this sport, too, there are no physical limitations: Figure skaters can range from 90 to 250 pounds. He does offer one caveat: Don't let the child take strenuous sessions at too young an age before the bone structure can stand the strains. (There are

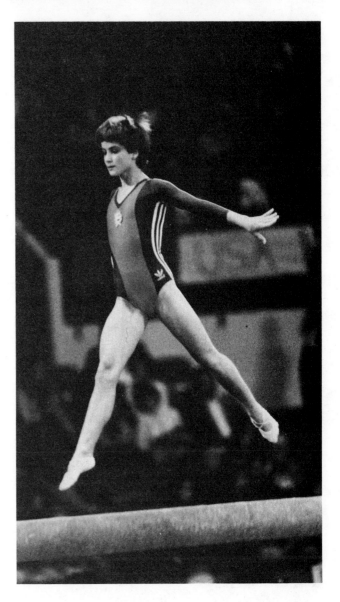

some strains on parents, too, who have to provide the transportation, costumes, equipment, and lessons, all of which cost.)

We've talked about age extension on the young side; there has also been age extension for women on the older side. Beth Anders has been the top scorer in women's field hockey for 14 years. At 31, still in Olympic competition, she says, "I want my team to be the best in the world!" And, of course, Billie Jean King, America's grande dame of sports is over 40 and still a top contender.

A note of caution to parents is sounded by Chris Rup of the Olympic sports medicine staff. She says youngsters should have the opportunity to participate in athletic activity whenever they show an interest: "Some youngsters don't respond well to organized sports. Their parents shouldn't try to force them. Let them come to athletics through play—learn to enjoy a game and develop general skill. Then if you find they have a particular talent or interest, encourage it. Don't hamper it with restrictions or demands. Give them an opportunity to play and have fun, and they'll come along naturally."

Chris feels parents are most helpful when they're encouraging. Some children need a lot of vocal support; others need physical support in the sense of having their parents in attendance at games and the knowledge that their parents are backing them up by providing transportation and encouragement. Above all, it's important to let the child be a good team player and not try to pressure the coach into giving the youngster a starring role.

Warm-up

As an adolescent athlete, you will have no trouble following the warm-up program outlined in Chapter V, page 101. Your youthful muscles will be slimmer but more supple than those of your seniors. We offer this counsel, however: If you come into this program without any previous training beyond casual school gym classes, you can start with about two-thirds the number of repetitions and work your way up to the indicated quota.

Stretching

In the following workout schedules for young women, stretching and flexibility are just as important as they are for adults. However, these exercises seem to come so easily for girls that they may want to zip through them in an offhand manner. Stretching is not a matter of speed, to get maximum benefit you must stretch slowly. Girls tend to be lacking in upper-arm strength. Concessions have been made in the method of doing push-ups from the floor and chin-ups from a hanging position. Start with doing one or two or three or as many as you can—then continue with the easier method. But keep building the muscles.

Aerobic Conditioning

You may jog, skip rope, do disco dancing to music, or dance with a long ribbon and baton (rhythmic gymnastics). Duration: not less than 10 minutes.

Alternately, you may ride a bike or use a stationary bike at a good steady clip for not less than 20 minutes.

Exercises for the Adolescent Female

These exercises are for the young female athlete. You're an athlete, and you can do most of the same exercises as well as boys and some even better. You should not do fewer than three workouts a week—four, if your schoolwork and other duties allow you the time.

Like all young athletes not in active competition, you will want to allow 48 hours between workouts. But you should try to do your stretching exercises and aerobics every day.

Set up an exercise schedule and keep a notebook to record the exercises you do. Work through all odd-numbered exercises on the odd-numbered days—days 1 and and 3—even-numbered exercises on even-numbered days—days 2 and 4—if you can manage four workouts. Remember, a workout should last approximately an hour and a half, including warm-up, stretching, aerobics, and cool-down. You'll find the exercises described and illustrated on page 60—95. All the warm-ups, stretching exercises, and aerobics outlined in this chapter should be part of every workout session. Then proceed to the muscle group conditioning.

1/
Push-ups *(See page 60.)*

Push up from a chair.

```
DAYS 1, 3

        Basic:     2 sets of 8 repetitions
     Improved:     3 sets of 6 repetitions
     Advanced:     3 sets of 7 repetitions
```

2/
Pump-ups *(See page 61.)*

```
DAYS 2, 4

        Basic:     2 sets of 3 repetitions
     Improved:     2 sets of 5·repetitions
     Advanced:     3 sets of 4 repetitions
```

3/
Chin-ups *(See page 62.)*

If you cannot pull yourself up, stand on a box, grasp
the bar, and slowly ease yourself down.

```
DAYS 1, 3

        Basic:     2 sets of 7 repetitions
     Improved:     2 sets of 7 repetitions
     Advanced:     3 sets of 5 repetitions
```

4/
French Curl *(See page 63.)*

You may use dumbbells or hand weights instead of the barbell.

DAYS 2, 4

Basic:	2 sets of 6 repetitions
Improved:	2 sets of 7 repetitions
Advanced:	3 sets of 5 repetitions

5/
Wrist Curl *(See page 64.)*

You may use dumbbells or hand weights instead of the barbell.

DAYS 1, 3

Basic:	2 sets of 6 repetitions
Improved:	3 sets of 5 repetitions
Advanced:	3 sets of 6 repetitions

6/
Bench Press *(See page 65.)*

You may use dumbbells or hand weights instead of the barbell.

DAYS 2, 4

Basic:	3 sets of 7 repetitions
Improved:	3 sets of 8 repetitions
Advanced:	3 sets of 8 repetitions

7/
Biceps Curl *(See page 66.)*

You may use dumbbells or hand weights instead of the barbell.

DAYS 1, 3	
Basic:	3 sets of 6 repetitions
Improved:	3 sets of 8 repetitions
Advanced:	3 sets of 8 repetitions

8/
Butterfly Swing *(See page 67.)*

DAYS 2, 4	
Basic:	3 sets of 4 repetitions
Improved:	3 sets of 5 repetitions
Advanced:	3 sets of 5 repetitions

9/
Ball Clutch *(See page 68.)*

DAYS 1, 3	
Basic:	3 sets of 10 repetitions
Improved:	6 sets of 10 repetitions
Advanced:	8 sets of 10 repetitions

10/
Towel Wring *(See page 68.)*

DAYS 2, 4

Basic:	2 sets of 4 repetitions
Improved:	3 sets of 6 repetitions
Advanced:	4 sets of 8 repetitions

The Mid Body

1/
Bent-knee Sit-ups *(See page 69.)*

DAYS 1, 3

Basic:	2 sets of 5 repetitions
Improved:	2 sets of 8 repetitions
Advanced:	3 sets of 6 repetitions

2/
Leg Lifts *(See page 70.)*

DAYS 2, 4

Basic:	1 set of 12 repetitions
Improved:	2 sets of 8 repetitions
Advanced:	3 sets of 6 repetitions

3/
Dumbbell Lifts *(See page 71.)*

DAYS 1, 3

Basic:	2 sets of 18 repetitions
Improved:	3 sets of 12 repetitions
Advanced:	3 sets of 12 repetitions

4/
Foot Lifts *(See page 72.)*

DAYS 2, 4

Basic:	2 sets of 9 repetitions
Improved:	2 sets of 10 repetitions
Advanced:	3 sets of 7 repetitions

5/
Lift-offs *(See page 73.)*

DAYS 1, 3

Basic:	2 sets of 12 repetitions
Improved:	3 sets of 9 repetitions
Advanced:	3 sets of 9 repetitions

6/
Round-up Twist *(See page 74.)*

DAYS 2, 4

Basic:	2 sets of 10 repetitions
Improved:	4 sets of 5 repetitions
Advanced:	4 sets of 7 repetitions

7/
Torso Torsion *(See page 76.)*

DAYS 1, 3

Basic:	1 set of 5 repetitions
Improved:	2 sets of 5 repetitions
Advanced:	2 sets of 10 repetitions

8/
Punting Practice *(See page 78.)*

DAYS 2, 4

Basic:	1 set of 5 repetitions
Improved:	2 sets of 8 repetitions
Advanced:	3 sets of 8 repetitions

9/
Weight Swing *(See page 80.)*

DAYS 1, 3

Basic:	2 sets of 12 repetitions
Improved:	3 sets of 12 repetitions
Advanced:	3 sets of 12 repetitions

10/
Towel Pull *(See page 82.)*

DAYS 2, 4

Basic:	2 sets of 9 repetitions
Improved:	2 sets of 10 repetitions
Advanced:	3 sets of 7 repetitions

The Lower Body

1/
No-chair Sit *(See page 83.)*

DAYS 1, 3

Basic:	2 sets of 12 repetitions
Improved:	3 sets of 12 repetitions
Advanced:	3 sets of 12 repetitions

2/
Hop-ups   *(See page 84.)*

DAYS 2, 4

Basic:	2 sets of 20 repetitions
Improved:	3 sets of 15 repetitions
Advanced:	3 sets of 15 repetitions

3/
Kneebends   *(See page 86.)*

DAYS 1, 3

Basic:	2 sets of 20 repetitions
Improved:	3 sets of 15 repetitions
Advanced:	3 sets of 15 repetitions

4/
Weighted Kneebends   *(See page 87.)*

DAYS 2, 4

Basic:	3 sets of 11 repetitions
Improved:	3 sets of 15 repetitions
Advanced:	3 sets of 15 repetitions

5/
Foot Lifts *(See page 88.)*

```
DAYS 1, 3

              Basic:    3 sets of 9 repetitions
           Improved:    3 sets of 10 repetitions
           Advanced:    3 sets of 10 repetitions
```

6/
Heel Dips *(See page 89.)*

```
DAYS 2, 4

              Basic:    2 sets of 12 repetitions
           Improved:    3 sets of 12 repetitions
           Advanced:    3 sets of 12 repetitions
```

7/
One-legged Heel Dips *(See page 89.)*

```
DAYS 1, 3

              Basic:    3 sets of 8 repetitions
           Improved:    3 sets of 10 repetitions
           Advanced:    3 sets of 10 repetitions
```

8/
Toe Curls *(See page 90.)*

DAYS 2, 4

Basic:	1 set of 5 repetitions
Improved:	2 sets of 5 repetitions
Advanced:	3 sets of 5 repetitions

9/
Leg Flutters *(See page 92.)*

DAYS 1, 3

Basic:	2 sets of 5 repetitions
Improved:	2 sets of 6 repetitions
Advanced:	2 sets of 6 repetitions

10/
Side-to-side Bounce *(See page 93.)*

DAYS 2, 4

Basic:	3 sets of 6 repetitions
Improved:	3 sets of 7 repetitions
Advanced:	3 sets of 9 repetitions

11/
Soleus Test and Flexion   *(See page 94.)*

DAYS 1, 3	
Basic:	2 sets of 5 repetitions
Improved:	2 sets of 10 repetitions
Advanced:	3 sets of 10 repetitions

12/
Climb-ups   *(See page 95.)*

DAYS 2, 4	
Basic:	2 sets of 18 repetitions
Improved:	3 sets of 15 repetitions
Advanced:	3 sets of 15 repetitions

Cool-down

Follow same routine as that given in Chapter IV for male athletes.

Maintenance

Earlier in this book, you read that women are gradually closing the sports gap with men. In past days, proper young ladies gave up their interest in sports and athletics at about the age of 14 or 15. Today, that's the age for the competitive young woman to get rolling in her chosen sport. In gymnastics and figure skating events, 14 and 15 are already the ages of champions. In other events, young women have set their sights on world class status.

How long will it be before women compete head-to-head against men? We can't answer that. But it may be your generation. And, in any case, you're proving that you certainly could compete against a lot of the male champions of a generation ago.

Sports is one of the most important arenas in which the battle for full women's equality is being waged. If you want to prove, as so many women assert, that you can be anything you want to be, the answer lies in getting the best possible coaching, continuing your body conditioning, following a sound, healthy diet—and getting out and showing the world!

CHAPTER VIII: CIRCUIT TRAINING—SUPER WORKOUT

You're an athlete. You've worked, you've trained. You've listened, you've learned, and you've practiced for long hours during long weeks. Now you want to move up the scale—to be an elite athlete, an Olympic aspirant, perhaps, possibly a world class contestant. You've had good coaching, and you're dedicated to your sport. Now let's hear some advice from coaches, trainers, and physiologists who are actually involved in Olympic competition.

"Quickness is the number-one trainable physiological attribute that determines whether an athlete will play at the highest level of competition." Those are the words of Jack Blatherwick, sports physiologist for the New York Rangers and also for the U.S. Olympic ice hockey team. "With Olympic-age athletes of 18 to 22, aerobic training is very important—for some players the most important form of training. And, of course, it's extremely important at the professional level. For ice hockey, we recommend sprint training—short sprints of 200 yards. If you're a young player trying to develop your skill, you've got to make endurance a part of it. Without endurance, a young player may lose up to half of his skill proficiency after as little as 30 seconds of extremely strenuous activity. Quickness, coordination, skill, and endurance are the qualities that make great players."

All coaches agree that an intensive training schedule is essential to competitive fitness. How intensive? In track events, Chris Rup of the Olympic sports medicine staff at the Olympic Training Center recommends about a two-hour workout. But if you're extremely strenuous about it, that would be a long time. She says, "In many cases, you can shorten a workout and get better quality. On the other hand, if you're in a team sport, two to two and one-half hours may be needed to shape up the players into working as a unit." In team sports and games, you may spend a good deal of time standing about or walking about between plays.

As for highly trained athletes in highly competitive situations, coaches may require seven days a week of training with double-day and triple-day workouts. Bob Beeten, associate director of sports medicine for the U.S. Olympic Training Center, believes in intensive training. "But," he says, "there is always a point of diminishing returns. Each athlete has to learn where that point is by what his body tells him. The average elite athlete can train up to four to six hours a day, though much of that may not be intensive, but rather at the skill level."

He agrees with other sports medicine authorities that very often a day or two a week away from intensive training can be advantageous so long as the athlete doesn't fritter away the time. Swimming or a long bike ride can be fun and useful in training and at the same time offer a change of scenery and a change of company.

Some Olympic trainers believe in year-round workouts, but many consider the psychological effect of such training as too heavy a mental grind for some athletes to bear. They suggest recreation and even participation in other sports during the off-season to allow the player to recover and recharge his enthusiasm, starting up again at a high level of intensity. But all agree that a certain amount of conditioning must go on year-round to maintain the cardiovascular system and muscle tone at a high level.

Jack Moser, also on the sports medicine staff, says, "You must distinguish between dedication to your sport and overintensity, which can cause burnout. Try to peak as you approach competition. Don't peak too early. The 'over-training syndrome' can cause you to go flat."

Steve Hornor, soccer trainer, says "You need to taper off in the last three days or so before an important contest to give your body time to recover." He also notes that Olympic coaches who demand seven-days-a-week training often use one or two of those days "to walk through things and talk through things." This is particularly true in strategic sports like soccer, hockey, and basketball.

In preparing for a contest, the competitive athlete will use the same warm-up, stretching, and aerobic exercises as we have outlined in Chapter IV. However, his aerobic training will be governed by the sports he's involved in. For running events, the 1½-mile (or equivalent) run is still a standard. But field and court sports require short bursts of speed combined with agility. Back-to-back 440-yard sprints are recommended for soccer and field hockey; 100-200 yard sprints for basketball and skiing; the 20-30, and 40-yard sprints for ice hockey, where blinding speed and change of pace over short time sequences is the goal.

But finally it comes back again to conditioning of the major muscle groups of the body. However, where the average active athlete is well served by the usual sets and repetitions, the competitive athlete must do "circuit" training. In the "circuit" workout, sets and whole exercise series are run back-to-back with no rest periods. The basic exercises are those already described but with new sequences.

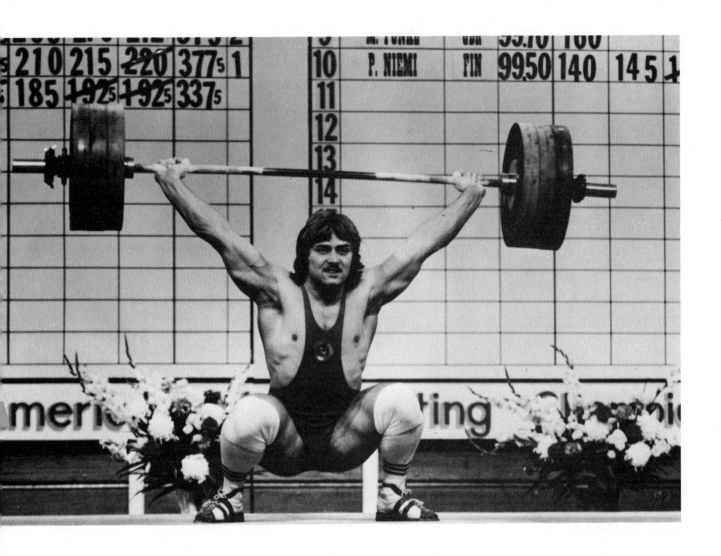

I wish that mental stuff would work for me, but I've just never found any substitute for hard work.
—Tommy Wigger, The Olympian, *June/July 1979*

Circuit Training

Routines for Week 1 of Circuit Training

Warm-ups, stretching, and aerobic conditioning described in Chapters IV and V except that adaptations to the contestant's particular sport are now necessary, particularly in aerobics and in warming up muscles to be most intensively used in competition.

CIRCUIT 1:

Perform Exercise 1 from Upper Body group, Exercise 1 from Mid Body group, and Exercise 1 from Lower Body group in sequence without resting.

CIRCUIT 2:

Same routine for Exercise 2 of each of the 3 muscle groups.

CIRCUIT 3:

Same routine for Exercise 3 of each of the muscle groups.

CIRCUIT 4:

Same routine for Exercise 4 of each group.

CIRCUIT 5:

Same routine for Exercise 5.

CIRCUIT 6:

Same routine for Exercise 6.

CIRCUIT 7:

Same routine for Exercise 7.

CIRCUIT 8:

Same routine for Exercise 8.

Routines for Weeks 2 and 3 of Circuit Training

These routines will duplicate week 1 training, but you will run one lap around the track between each circuit. If no track or running space is available, run in place, skip rope, or use a stationary bike for 30 seconds between circuits.

Routines for Weeks 4 and 5 of Circuit Training

Routines for week 4 and 5 will duplicate weeks 2 and 3, but you will add a total of 5 repetitions to each exercise. Thus, if an exercise calls for 5 sets of 5 reps, you will do 5 sets of 6 reps. If the exercise calls for 2 sets of 20 reps, you will do 1 set of 22 and 1 set of 23. Total added reps for each exercise must not equal fewer than 5 (6 is acceptable).

Routines for Weeks 6 and 7 of Circuit Training

Routines for these weeks will duplicate weeks 2 and 3 but now you will run two laps between circuits or perform 45 seconds of running in place, rope jumping, or bike pedaling between circuits.

Routines for Weeks 8 and 9 of Circuit Training

Routines for these weeks will duplicate weeks 2 and 3, but now you will add a total of 10 reps to each exercise. Continue two laps or 45 seconds of aerobics between circuits.

Routines for Weeks 10, 11, and 12 of Circuit Training

Routines for these weeks will duplicate weeks 8 and 9, but now you will run three laps of take a full minute of aerobic running in place, rope skipping, or bike pedaling between circuits.

Cool-down

Since the exercise activity in circuit training is intended for the competitive athlete who is preparing for an event, it is considerably more intensive than the training for the average active athlete. Cool-down should therefore be extended to permit more stretching. Particularly important will be the stretching exercise for Achilles' tendon (exercise 2, page 51), the Hamstring Limber-up (exercise 1, page 50) and torso and shoulder stretching (exercises 5 and 6, pages 54 and 55). Always bear in mind that stretching during cool-down is virtually as important as during warm-up.

Specific Variations

If you are in active competition, your coach or trainer will probably add specific exercises for the muscle groups important to your sport or event. (See Chapter X for a reference table on this subject.) If you are training on your own, you'd be well advised to find the best gym or training facility available to you, particularly one with Nautilus, Universal, or CAM II equipment or combinations of these machines. The advantage of these machines is that they provide full-range exercise, which includes unrestricted speed of movement, rotary-form movement, and automatically variable resistance, which weights and simple exercise machines do not. They also place far greater emphasis on negative work (lowering the weight after lifting it), which should be done at half the speed of positive work (lifting the weight). Physiol-

ogists are placing increasing importance on this negative aspect of working with resistance machines or weights.

The circuit training routines have been designed to provide overload conditioning. The body can only approach maximum efficiency through overload training. This does not mean working out to the point of exhaustion; at that point you are in imminent danger of injury. Overload training means pushing to the absolute limit of your muscle abilities, increasing the load gradually so that you are regularly exceeding your preceding best effort. In exercises requiring the barbell, for example, slowly add weight to it as you progress in your training.

If you cannot get through all the circuits without rest, then use the interval method of breaking up the workout program with rest intervals. But try to shorten the intervals gradually and finally eliminate them.

Of course, you're going to feel anxious, possibly even depressed before your event. This is common to most athletes—the fear that they're not going to measure up to their best capabilities. Coaches no longer believe they have to "psych up" their players in the famous tradition attributed to Knute Rockne. As Beth Anders of the U.S. Olympics hockey team and leading scorer for 14 years puts it, "My biggest problem is staying relaxed before a game. Beginning a full hour before the start, I just concentrate on relaxing. I think of what I have to do, and I mentally rehearse all the motions I'll be going through. I don't get mad or tense. Calmness is the key."

The secret to winning does not lie in playing above your head; it lies in the amount and kind of training you have under your belt.

My records will be broken. When I'm forty-five, there'll be kids in high school dual meets who'll be jumping beyond my American record. But if I can leave behind something so that athletes will stay in the sport longer because they saw Dwight Stones jumping until he was thirty and having a personal record when he was thirty, that makes me feel good because I think I'm partially responsible for it.
—Dwight Stones, six-time U.S. high-jump champion

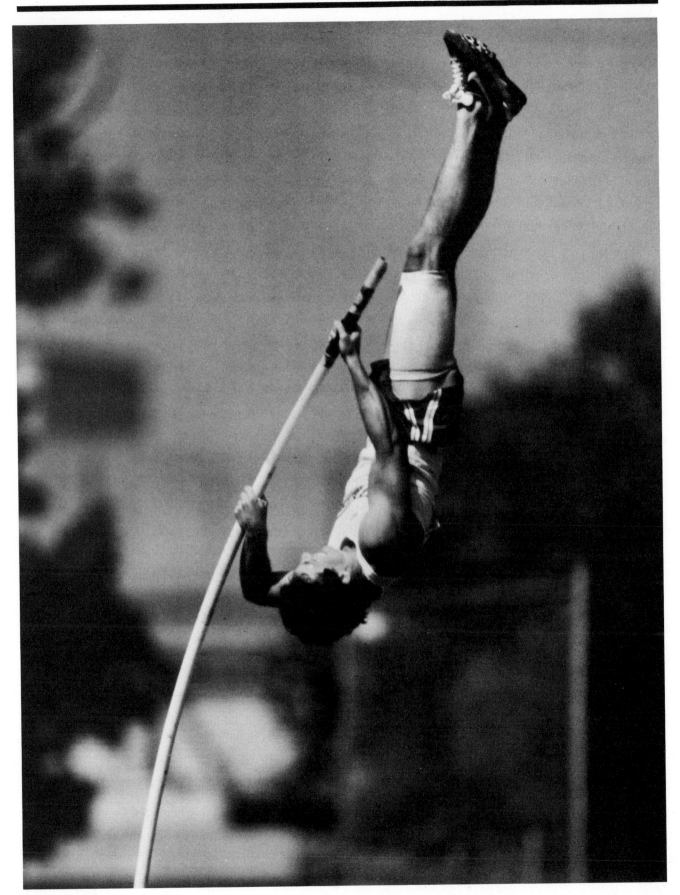

CHAPTER IX: DIET AND NUTRITION FOR THE COMPETITIVE ATHLETE

One of the reasons that we are healthier and longer-lived than ever before in history—and that today's athletes are constantly establishing new records—is that we have learned a great deal about nutrition and the human body.

The idea that "we are what we eat" goes back to the early part of this century. In those days, to the burly athlete and his coach, this meant that if you ate a lot of red meat, you developed big muscles and improved the quality of your blood. To today's sophisticated sports nutritionists, eating a heavy meat diet is a thing of the past. Healthy athletes eat what healthy people anywhere eat—a balanced diet of what we know as the basic four food groups: meat and protein sources, dairy, grain, and fruits and vegetables. Contained within the various combinations of these four food groups are indispensable vitamins and minerals. Finally, of course, everybody requires water.

To most adults, the word *diet* connotes a weight-loss regimen. Even professional athletes tend to go "out of training" and "off their diets" when their season ends, then go back on their diets and in training to slim down and prepare for the new season. The successful competitive athlete never goes out of training or off his diet—it has become a lifestyle, though he or she obviously intensifies training before an important game or event. He or she is concerned with "weight management," or maintenance of body weight at an ideal level, increasing calories if below the ideal weight and decreasing them if above.

SWLG Corporation's Officially Licensed Fitness Program of the XIV Olympic Winter Games, which program is marketed under the name EASY AS 1 2 3™ WEIGHT MANAGEMENT SYSTEM, offers an alternative to fad diets and "magic" weight loss promotions, which should be avoided at all costs. This system was devised after extensive research in nutrition, behavior modification, and exercise, and was evaluated by a professional advisory board of top medical and nutritional experts. More than 150 diet plans were studied, and their common success and failure factors noted. The EASY AS 1 2 3™ WEIGHT MANAGEMENT SYSTEM includes not only individual computerized daily menus but also exercise and behavior modification techniques and tapes. The following are some of the principles of the plan.

Weight should not be altered by more than 4 percent of your present body weight per month. In other words, if you weigh 150 pounds, don't try to put on or take off more than 6 pounds (4 percent) in 30 days. The sensible way to control weight is by adding to or subtracting from the number of calories in your normal daily food intake while still maintaining a balanced selection from the four basic food groups.

A well-balanced diet contains about 50 percent of the calories in carbohydrates, up to 20 percent in protein, and up to 30 percent in fats.

Carbohydrate foods include breads, cereals, grains, starchy vegetables such as potatoes, corn, peas, and beans, plus fruits of all types, including apples, bananas, pears, and pineapples. Carbohydrates are emphasized in a healthy, athletic diet because they break down easily into glucose, a simple sugar that is the primary source of quick and efficient energy used by the body.

Proteins and fats are also an energy source, but they are harder to digest than carbohydrates, and there is no evidence that they are in any way superior to carbohydrates as an energy source. In addition, meats—particularly pork and beef—are often accompanied by objectionable amounts of saturated fats. For this reason, lean cuts are to be preferred, and meats should always be well trimmed. Weight lifters, shot-putters, hammer throwers, and other extremely active athletes for whom a heavily muscled body is important require additional calories for energy, as well as increased nutrients, including protein. These needs are met by increasing the quantity of a well-balanced diet in all of the basic four food categories.

High-fat foods include dairy products such as milk, butter, cream, margarine, and eggs, along with nuts, avocados, peanut butter, cooking oils, and, of course, meats. The American Heart Association and many nutritionists caution against excessive fat in the diet. Excessive fat in the diet increases the cholesterol level in the blood, which may lead to arteriosclerosis, a contributing factor in heart disease. Dietary fat is not directly related to body fat. Although dietary fat is a concentrated energy source, excessive calories from any food source (protein, carbohydrates, and fats) will be stored as body fat. The optimum percentage of body fat for a normal man is 12 to 16 percent; for a long-distance runner, it may be as low as 4 to 8 percent; for a football player in the line, as high as 18 percent. Body fat percentages run higher in women—on the average, about 22 percent. In a female distance runner, the percentage rarely goes below 12 percent.

A good breakfast will usually be rich in carbohydrates, including breads and cereals. Although many of today's white breads have been enriched with vitamins and minerals lost in the milling process, dark breads are, in general, richer in whole grains than are lighter ones. Presweetened cereals should be limited. As for cereals that promise you 100 percent of your daily minimum requirement of vitamins and minerals, no fault is to be found except in the price. A well-balanced diet should supply you with more than 100 percent of your daily requirements. If

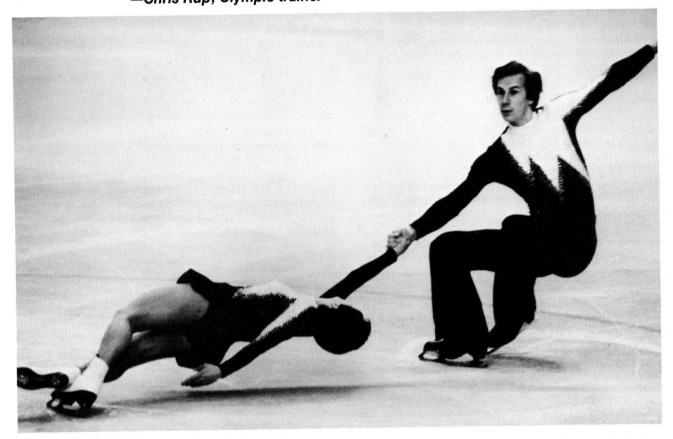

you have any doubt that your intake of vitamins and minerals is adequate, you will probably do your body no harm by taking a recommended vitamin supplement. Check with your doctor on this. Excessive intake of some vitamin and mineral supplements may cause deficiencies in other vitamins and minerals. Niacin and riboflavin, for example, are depleted by heavy doses of thiamine, and heavy intake of vitamin A and D tablets may lead to toxic symptoms such as headaches. Athletes have a tendency to be almost superstitious about taking certain special diet supplements simply because some friend recommended them. Your best friend in recommending such supplements should be your doctor or nutritionist.

One category of foods that is difficult to overdo is fruits and vegetables. Plentifully enriched with vitamins and minerals, satisfying to the taste, and high in the fiber that aids digestion while providing low-calorie bulk, fresh fruits and vegetables have been steadily increasing in importance in the diet of modern man. Credit for this may go back to the British navy for first learning that the scourge of scurvy, so often encountered on H.M.S. vessels, could easily be avoided by adding a plentiful supply of long-last-

ing limes to the ships' food stores. The appellation "limey," applied to the British sailor, may have started as a taunt, but their superior training and nutrition enabled the "limeys" to rule the seas during the great centuries of ocean commerce.

Until recently, many active athletes expressed an irrational prejudice against the drinking of water. How often have we seen boxers or football players gulp a mouthful of water and then spit it out as if it were poisonous? New knowledge of the body processes has changed all that, and now it is common practice for the marathon runner, the distance bike rider, and the cross-country skier to sip freely from a water flask—for the body is not only lubricated and cooled by fluids, it is largely composed of fluid. During strenuous exercise, the body may lose four to five pounds of fluid in an hour. The well-conditioned body does not store surplus fluid as it might store surplus fat or glucose against a severe drain. Nor does it "toughen you up" (as some coaches used to think) to hold down on fluids after an intensive workout. Neither does the normal body need salt tablets to replenish salt lost in perspiration, as was formerly believed. The "basic four" diet should provide all the salt the body needs to keep up its supply during and after strenuous activity.

Timing of workouts in relation to meals is important. You should not engage in rigorous exercise for at least an hour after eating breakfast or lunch and an hour and a half after eating dinner. If you work out before breakfast—or, for that matter, anytime—it's a good idea to have a glass of water or some diluted fruit juice before exercising. This is particularly important during hot weather.

Starting your day with a well-balanced breakfast is always desirable. During fitness training, it provides a sound energy foundation for your athletic demands. Be sure to include at least one good source of vitamin C such as strawberries, tomatoes, orange juice, grapefruit, cantaloupe, and most berries. B-complex vitamins, which are essential to the balanced diet, are derived from whole-grain breads and cereals, beef, pork, liver, dried beans, peas, soybeans, peanuts, eggs, milk, and dark-green leafy vegetables. Your daily diet should also include important minerals. Sodium, one such essential diet element, is readily found in milk, eggs, meat, poultry, fish, spinach, beets, celery, chard, and, of course, salt. Potassium, another necessary mineral, is found in meats, poultry, fish, bananas, potatoes, tomatoes, carrots, celery, oranges, and grapefruit.

An individual who is on a low-cholesterol regimen should consume less red meat, fewer eggs, and more fish, chicken, and turkey for variety. Limit lobster, shrimp, oysters, clams, and crabs, because they contain high amounts of cholesterol. Also limit whole milk, butter, and high-fat cheeses in favor of skim milk, low-fat cheeses, and margarine. Plain yogurt is a preferable alternative to ice cream or other rich, sugary desserts.

Olympic athletes and nutrition experts are frequently asked what should be eaten before an important game or event. The technique of carbohydrate loading is advocated by some coaches, trainers, and athletes to enhance endurance during a competitive event. The purpose is to supersaturate the muscles with glycogen to be used during the competition. There are two phases involved. Phase I, the depletion phase, starts four to seven days prior to the event. Intake of complex carbohydrates is reduced to approximately 100 grams per day, depending on body weight. Phase II, the supersaturation phase, begins one to three days before the day of the event, at which time complex carbohydrate intake is emphasized. A minimum of 250 to 525 grams of carbohydrate is needed during each day of Phase II. For short events, Phase I can be eliminated, and Phase II alone will supply the glycogen required for short events, but will not "supersaturate" glycogen stores.

Carbohydrate loading is generally not recommended for the average athlete. The diet can be nutritionally inadequate if not properly planned. It should be used sparingly (not more than two or three times per year), and is not recommended for persons with cardiovascular disease or diabetes. All athletes should consult with their doctors before attempting to "carbohydrate load." In any case, on the day of an event, meals should be lighter than usual, and nothing should be eaten for at least two hours before competing, to allow significant digestion to take place. No modern adviser recommends a candy bar for a quick jolt of energy just before going into action. There is evidence that eating candy before competition actually *lowers* your available sugar reserves! You should be safe if you rely minimally on meat protein (not more than 15 percent of caloric intake) and heavily (85 percent) on breads, cereals, fruits, vegetables, and milk products in preparation for competition.

After the event, there are a variety of thirst quenchers suggested with a variety of opinions as to which is best, such as water, diluted fruit juice, and electrolite replacement beverages, or, as recommended by at least one sports physician, a glass of beer. Stay away from icy cold beverages when the body is overheated.

If you are looking for weight stability, the EASY AS 1 2 3™ WEIGHT MANAGEMENT SYSTEM offers a sensible array of choices for your daily menu, with tasty substitutions for foods for which you've never been able to develop a taste.

To maintain your weight, you need to take in a certain amount of calories. This number of calories is called your "balance point." If you want to lose weight, you must take in fewer calories than your balance point. To gain weight, you must take in more calories than your balance point. The number of calories arrived at by either of these adjustments is called your "diet base." As you lose or gain weight, your balance point will change. You must recalculate your balance point once a month to compensate for these changes.

This weight-control plan is predicated upon the formula that if you are a relatively active person, you need about 14 to 16 calories a day per pound of body mass to keep your weight stable. During periods of high activity, you will need 16 to 18 calories per pound, and during periods of inactivity no more than 12 to 14 calories per pound of body weight per day. For example: During periods of normal activity, a person weighing 130 pounds would require 130 x 14 or 1,820 calories a day to maintain steady weight. Fewer calories would result in weight loss; more than 1,820 calories will result in weight gain for most people.

The dietary and nutritional aspect of the EASY AS 1 2 3™ WEIGHT MANAGEMENT SYSTEM is a personal computerized program with health benefits that can last a lifetime. It is based on menus of variable caloric intake designated as One-Day, Two-Day, and Three-Day menus called Vari-Diet menus. The Vari-Diet menus are for 30 days and are based on each individual's own weight and activity level. Each individual's Vari-Diet menus are provided in a computer printout called a Comp-U-Plan.

There are two advantages to the One-Day, Two-Day, Three-Day Vari-Diet pattern. First, the typical American does not consume a constant quantity of food day after day. For example, food consumption tends to be higher on weekends and special occasions; therefore, the EASY AS 1 2 3™ WEIGHT MANAGEMENT SYSTEM is designed to fit the American lifestyle.

Second, by having a variety of three calorie levels, the body is unable to adjust to a set calorie level. This helps to prevent undesirable weight plateaus that can occur when following a rigid diet regimen of one constant caloric level. Menus indicated by the 1 2 3 Vari-Diet Pattern Selector may be arranged on a calendar to plan for the higher calorie days (Three-Days) on weekends and special occasions when you expect to be consuming more calories. The lower calorie days (One- and Two-Days) may be scheduled during the week when the tendency is to eat lighter meals or to be less active.

NOTE: The Comp-U-Plan and Vari-Diet examples given in this chapter are only general examples for illustration. They are not meant as strict guidelines for designing your own nutritional program, because many other personal variables must be taken into account for a safe and effective program. The calculations are complex and difficult to do manually, and there is room for error if done manually, which is why EASY AS 1 2 3 uses a sophisticated computer. In addition, this is only a part of the entire EASY AS 1 2 3™ WEIGHT MANAGEMENT SYSTEM. For full details, you may contact EASY AS 1 2 3 at 4101 Perimeter Center Drive, Suite 300, Oklahoma City, OK 73112 or phone 1-800-654-6770 or 405-947-7621.

Menus are composed of portions called "food values." The caloric content of one food value for each food group is as follows:

1 food value of: Protein   70 calories

1 food value of: Breads and cereals   70 calories
1 food value of: Milk and dairy products   100 calories
1 food value of: Fruit   80 calories
1 food value of: Vegetable   50 calories
1 food value of: Fat   50 calories

The amount of each food on the food value table corresponds to *one* food value in the diet. In other words, if your Three-Day calls for two food values of protein for breakfast, refer to the protein chart and select, for example, one portion of cottage cheese and one medium egg. The combination of the two will satisfy the requirements for two food values of protein.

The Vari-Diet Pattern Selector, page 166, gives the balance point with the variations in eating levels. As the balance point increases, the One-, Two-, and Three-Day segments shift into higher caloric menus (the One-Days are the lowest calorie level on the left, the Two-Days are indicated by the middle number, and the number of Three-Days are on the right). There are menu patterns for each caloric level following this Vari-Diet Pattern Selector. As weight is lost or gained, the balance point changes and must be recalculated monthly.

To use the Vari-Diet Pattern Selector, round off your balance point to the nearest 100 calories. Find the resulting figure in the left-hand column of the pattern selector. Directly to the right of that figure are three numbers. These numbers refer to the number of days in a month that you should use at that calorie level menu pattern, which is indicated by the heading in that column, if you want to stay at your current weight (see page 167 for menu patterns).

If you want to lose weight, you must subtract calories from your balance point. The figure you arrive at by such a subtraction is called your "diet base" figure. As in the example above, you would find your diet base figure in the left-hand column of the pattern selector and go to the right to find the number of One-, Two-, and Three-days necessary to lose the weight. The same procedure is done if you want to gain weight, except that you *add* calories to your balance point.

This is only a basic explanation of how a person could develop a safe and effective weight-loss or weight-gain program. There are other, more complex calculations that also have to be made in order to arrive at a tailor-made program for you.

(Keep in mind that One-Days in the menu will have the fewest calories, Two-Days have more, and Three-Days have the greatest number of calories.)

Vari-Diet Pattern Selector

(Number of days per month at various calorie levels)

Diet Base or Balance Point	1000 Calories	1500 Calories	2020 Calories	2770 Calories	3470 Calories	4200 Calories	4970 Calories
1000	30						
1100	26	2	2				
1200	21	6	3				
1300	17	5	5				
1400	13	10	7				
1500	10	10	10				
1600	6	12	12				
1700	1	16	13				
1800		16	12	2			
1900		13	13	4			
2000		10	14	6			
2100		7	15	8			
2200		4	16	10			
2300		1	17	12			
2400			17	11	2		
2500			14	13	3		
2600			10	17	3		
2700			6	21	3		
2800			2	25	3		
2900			1	22	7		
3000				21	8	1	
3100				18	10	2	
3200				16	10	4	
3300				12	13	5	
3400				9	15	6	
3500				7	15	8	
3600				5	15	10	
3700				3	15	12	
3800					16	14	
3900					13	16	1
4000					10	18	2
4100					6	22	2
4200					4	22	3
4300					2	22	6
4400					1	20	9
4500					1	16	13
4600					4	7	19
4700					3	5	22
4800					3	1	26
4900					1	1	28

Menu Patterns
Calorie Level Menu Patterns

1,000 calories

Breakfast	Lunch	Dinner
1 protein	2 protein	2 protein
1 bread	1 bread	1 fruit
1 milk	1 milk	1 Class A or
1 fruit	1 fruit	1 Class B vegetable
	1 Class A vegetable	
	1 fat	

1,500 calories

Breakfast	Lunch	Dinner
1 protein	2 protein	2 protein
1 bread	2 bread	1 bread
1 milk	1 milk	1 milk
1 fruit	1 fruit	2 fruit
	1 Class A vegetable	1 Class A vegetable
	1 Class B vegetable	1 Class B vegetable
	1 fat	

2,020 calories

Breakfast	Lunch	Dinner
1 protein	2 protein	3 protein
1 bread	2 bread	2 bread
1 milk	1 milk	1 milk
2 fruit	2 fruit	2 fruit
	2 Class A vegetables	2 Class A vegetables
	1 Class B vegetable	1 Class B vegetable
	1 fat	1 fat

2,770 calories

Breakfast	Lunch	Dinner
2 protein	2 protein	4 protein
3 bread	4 bread	3 bread
1 milk	2 milk	1 milk
2 fruit	3 fruit	2 fruit
1 fat	2 Class A vegetables	2 Class A vegetables
	2 Class B vegetables	2 Class B vegetables
	1 fat	1 fat

3,470 calories

Breakfast	Lunch	Dinner
2 protein	4 protein	4 protein
3 bread	4 bread	3 bread
2 milk	2 milk	2 milk
3 fruit	3 fruit	3 fruit
2 fat	3 Class A vegetables	2 Class A vegetables
	2 Class B vegetables	3 Class B vegetables
	2 fat	1 fat

4,200 calories

Breakfast	Lunch	Dinner
2 protein	5 protein	5 protein
4 bread	4 bread	4 bread
3 milk	3 milk	3 milk
3 fruit	3 fruit	3 fruit
2 fat	3 Class A vegetables	2 Class A vegetables
	3 Class B vegetables	3 Class B vegetables
	3 fat	2 fat

4,970 calories

Breakfast	Lunch	Dinner
2 protein	6 protein	6 protein
4 bread	5 bread	5 bread
3 milk	3 milk	3 milk
4 fruit	4 fruit	4 fruit
2 fat	4 Class A vegetables	4 Class A vegetables
	4 Class B vegetables	4 Class B vegetables
	3 fat	2 fat

Some meals, especially those in higher caloric levels, may be too bulky to eat at one time. If this occurs, food values may be saved for in-between-meal or evening snacks.

Food Value Table

Each item below equals one food value in the above diet plan. Note that one type of food may be freely substituted for another type of food as long as they are both from the same food grouping and are exchanged food value for food value. For example, one slice of bread may be substituted for one-half an English muffin.

Bread Values

Bread—1 ounce or slice
Cereal, cold unsugared—1 cup
Cereal, cooked—½ cup
Grits, cooked—½ cup
Muffin, English—one-half

Milk Values

Buttermilk—1 cup
Low-fat milk—¾ cup
Skim milk—1¼ cup
Lowfat yogurt, plain—¾ cup

Protein Values

Cheese, cottage (2 percent fat)—3 ounces
*Cheese, hard—¾ ounce
* Egg—1 medium
Fish—1 ⅓ ounces, cooked
Chicken (no skin)—1 ½ ounces, cooked
Liver—1 ounce, cooked
Tuna, water-packed—2 ounces, drained
** Beef, ham, lamb, pork—1 ounce, cooked

* Limit 4 per week
** Limit 3 per week

Fruit Values

Apple—1 medium
Banana—1 small (6")
Berries—1 cup
Cantaloupe—½ small
Grapes—¾ cup
Grapefruit—1 medium
Orange—1 medium
Peach—2 medium
Pear—¾ medium
Juices, unsweetened—½ cup

Vegetable Values, Class A

Asparagus—1 cup
Broccoli—1 cup
Cabbage (cooked)—1 ½ cups
Cauliflower—2 cups
Celery—10 small stalks
Cucumber—1 medium
Leafy greens, lettuce—2 cups
Onions, raw—1 ¼ cup
Peppers, green—1 cup
Pickles, dill—4 medium
Radishes—1 cup
Squash, summer—1 ½ cups
Turnips—1 ½ cups
Zucchini—1 ½ cups

Vegetable Values, Class B

Artichokes—1 medium
Beets—1 cup
Brussels sprouts—8 each
Carrots—1 cup
Eggplant—1 cup
Okra (small)—16 each
Onion, cooked—1 cup
Parsnips—½ cup
Peas—½ cup
Rutabaga—¾ cup
Squash, winter—⅓ cup
Tomatoes, medium—1 ½ each
Green beans—2 cups
Corn—¼ cup

Women and men, and certainly young athletes in school, often carry heavy schedules and may be tempted to skip breakfast or lunch. The best advice is—don't! If you're pressed for time, here are two Quickie Meals in a Glass that can be prepared in a blender; however, these recipes may be only part of what you personally require for a meal and should not be used continuously as a substitute.

Orange Shake

    ½ cup unsweetened orange juice
    ½ cup plain yogurt
    1 raw egg
    5 or 6 ice cubes

Banana Smoothie

    1 very ripe banana
    ⅓ cup nonfat dry milk
    1 raw egg
    ½ teaspoon vanilla extract
    6 ice cubes

Combine ingredients in a blender until smooth. Serve with a piece of toast for a balanced breakfast or other meal.

Active athletic people, just like everyone else, eat in restaurants from time to time. This need not be a challenge to your fitness diet nor require a severe infraction of it. Plan in advance on the food values you will want and the approximate caloric content of each. The EASY AS 1 2 3 plan suggests that you call the restaurant ahead of time and explain that you're on a training or special diet and what your requirements are. Most restaurant staffs prove to be highly cooperative. EASY AS 1 2 3 also recommends that you enlist the support of your waiter or waitress by explaining your needs and the reason for them. This way you assure your servers that you're not a picky eater finding fault with the menu; instead, you turn them into cooperative allies.

Snack foods and fast-food restaurants are so much a part of all our lives that it is useless to tell you to avoid them totally. The main problem with snack foods is that many are often too rich in fats and are prepared by frying, as in the case of potato chips. Other snack foods tend to be too high in sugar and salt content. If you're careful, you'll check the label and forgo those high in fat, sugar, or salt. You should remember that the ingredients are listed in the order of their proportionate part of the total (in other words, the first item listed is the main ingredient).

Fast-food restaurants have come a long way (and are still progressing) in catering to health-food-minded eaters. Try to select those with salad bars, being careful to avoid rich dressings. And remember that although "juicy" hamburgers may look more succulent, drier ones have less fat. Broiling is always preferred to frying.

As to alcohol, your conscience must be your guide. Today, mineral water with a slice of lemon or lime is a fashionable and agreeable drink at cocktail parties. If you must drink alcohol, do so in moderation. Wines are preferable to hard liquor. You can reduce the amount of wine consumed during an evening by mixing it with soda or seltzer for a "spritzer"—a quite acceptable drink in any social setting. Seltzer is becoming generally preferred to club soda because of its lower sodium content.

Indicated nutrition values are based on the U.S. Department of Agriculture, Handbook Number 8; U.S. Department of Agriculture Handbook of the Nutritional Contents of Foods; and National Research Council Recommended Dietary Allowances, Ninth Edition.

There's probably some kid out there we've never even heard of who's going to end up being a top prospect for the Olympic squad.
—Bobby Knight, Olympic basketball coach

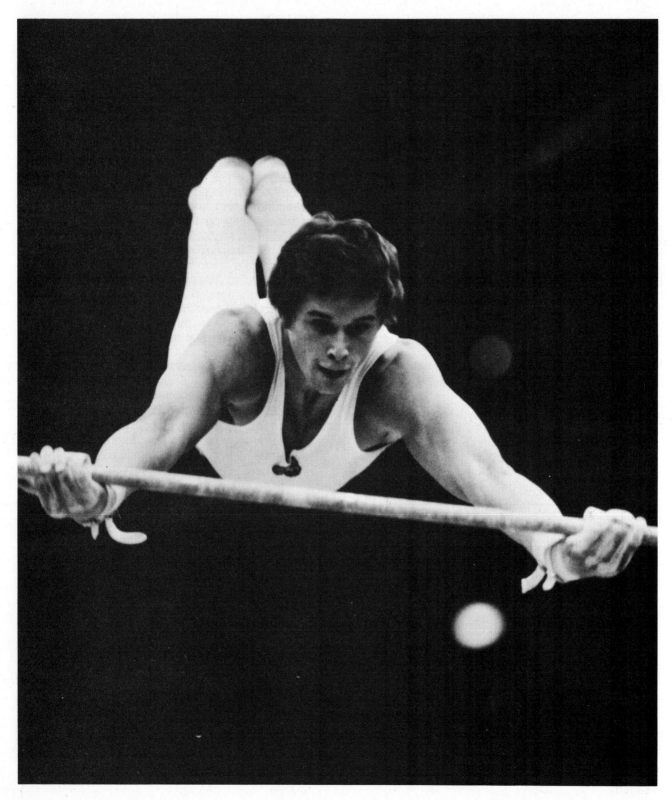

CHAPTER X: SPECIALIZED CONDITIONING FOR INDIVIDUAL SPORTS

There are two general ways of training for a specific sport or event:

1. Keep on repeating the game or event over and over; for instance, playing two or three sets of tennis every morning and another two or three sets every afternoon or getting out on the field and putting the shot for two or three hours at a time or skiing all day, day after day during the season, on all kinds of slopes or slalom courses.

2. Recognizing the main muscle groups and associated muscle groups that are involved in your activity and actively working to develop them to maximum efficiency, along with aerobic workouts for sports where endurance is important—plus regular practice in your sport or event.

Olympic trainers and athletes are virtually unanimous in preferring the second training regimen. Over and over, they emphasize that the achievement of record-breaking performances has been attained by deeper knowledge of the body's physiological potentials and more effective training techniques for fine-tuning it.

The following pages tabulate major sport groups and event groups and analyze the kind of training exercises that will help most in improving your performance standards when combined with actual practice in sports activity itself.

In performing the exercises, it's important to hone them to your needs. Soccer and ice hockey require speed and agility. Slow jogging and heavy weight-lifting will not satisfy those needs. Pace up the exercises where your sport requires quickness.

The athletic activities covered below include most of the Olympic events.

The first column rates the kinds of demands made on the body by the sport or event: XXX is most demanding; XX is less demanding; X is still lower. The muscle group emphasis is rated in the second column, indicating which groups need the most conditioning, and the exercises recommended for this conditioning are listed in the third column, referring back to Chapters IV and V; UP indicates Upper Body exercises; MB means Mid Body, and LB refers to Lower Body.

The regular warm-up and stretching exercises must precede special exercise routines. Where strong emphasis is laid upon a given muscle group, gradually build up the sets and reps to a point beyond the demands that would be made in a game! The amount of aerobic conditioning should be proportionate to that indicated in the Body Demands column.

Body Demands		Muscle Group Emphasis		Recommended Exercises

RACQUET GAMES

Tennis

Body Demands		Muscle Group Emphasis		Recommended Exercises
Aerobic Endurance	XX	Upper Body	XXX	UP 3,4,5,6,7
Power	X	Mid Body	XX	MB 1,2,4,5,6,9
Stamina	XX	Lower Body	XX	LB 1,2,3,6,9,10
Speed	XXX			
Flexibility	XX			

Racquet Ball (also Squash and Paddle Ball)

Body Demands		Muscle Group Emphasis		Recommended Exercises
Aerobic Endurance	XX	Upper Body	XX	UP 3,4,5,6,7
Power	X	Mid Body	XX	MB 2,4,5,6,9
Stamina	XX	Lower Body		LB 3,6,9,10
Speed	XX			
Flexibility	XX			

171

TEAM SPORTS

Basketball

Body Demands		Muscle Group Emphasis		Recommended Exercises
Aerobic Endurance	XXX	Upper Body	XX	UP 1,2,3,5
Power	XX	Mid Body	X	MB 1,4,5,9
Stamina	XX	Lower Body	XXX	LB 2,3,4,6
Speed	XXX			
Flexibility	XXX			

Volley Ball

Body Demands		Muscle Group Emphasis		Recommended Exercises
Aerobic Endurance	XX	Upper Body	XXX	UP 1,3,4,7,8
Power	X	Mid Body	X	MB 1,2,4,5,6
Stamina	XX	Lower Body	XX	LB 1,2,3,4,6
Speed	XX			
Flexibility	XXX			

Soccer

Body Demands		Muscle Group Emphasis		Recommended Exercises
Aerobic Endurance	XXX	Upper Body	X	UP 3,7,8
Power	XX	Mid Body	XX	MB 1,2,4,6,10
Stamina	XX	Lower Body	XXX	LB 1,2,4,5,6
Speed	XXX			
Flexibility	XXX			

Water Polo

Body Demands		Muscle Group Emphasis		Recommended Exercises
Aerobic Endurance	XX	Upper Body	XXX	UP 1,2,3,5,7
Power	XXX	Mid Body	XX	MB 1,2,4,5,6
Stamina	XXX	Lower Body	XX	LB 1,2,4,9,12
Speed	XXX			
Flexibility	XX			

Ice Hockey

Body Demands		Muscle Group Emphasis		Recommended Exercises
Aerobic Endurance	XXX	Upper Body	XX	UP 1,2,3,4,5,7
Power	XX	Mid Body	XX	MB 1,2,4,5,6
Stamina	XXX	Lower Body	XXX	LB 1,2,3,4,6,12
Speed	XXX			
Flexibility	XXX			

Rowing

Body Demands		Muscle Group Emphasis		Recommended Exercises
Aerobic Endurance	XXX	Upper Body	XXX	UP 1,2,3,4,6,7
Power	XXX	Mid Body	XXX	MB 1,2,3,5,9,10
Stamina	XXX	Lower Body	XX	LB 2,3,4,6,9,12
Speed	X			
Flexibility	X			

Field Hockey

Body Demands		Muscle Group Emphasis		Recommended Exercises
Aerobic Endurance	XXX	Upper Body	XX	UP 1,2,3,5,7
Power	XX	Mid Body	XX	MB 1,2,4,5,6
Stamina	XXX	Lower Body	XXX	LB 1,2,3,10,12
Speed	XX			
Flexibility	XXX			

Yachting

Body Demands		Muscle Group Emphasis		Recommended Exercises
Aerobic Endurance	X	Upper Body	XX	UP 2,3,4,6,7,8
Power	XX	Mid Body	X	MB 1,3,4,9,10
Stamina	XX	Lower Body	X	LB 3,6,9,12
Speed	X			
Flexibility	X			

SWIMMING EVENTS

Racing

Body Demands		Muscle Group Emphasis		Recommended Exercises
Aerobic Endurance	XXX	Upper Body	XXX	UP 1,3,4,6,7
Power	XX	Mid Body	XX	MB 2,4,6,9,10
Stamina	XX	Lower Body	XX	LB 1,2,5,9
Speed	XXX			
Flexibility	XX			

Synchronous Swimming

Body Demands		Muscle Group Emphasis		Recommended Exercises
Aerobic Endurance	XX	Upper Body	XX	UP 1,2,3,5,7
Power	X	Mid Body	XX	MB 1,5,6,9,10
Stamina	XXX	Lower Body	XX	LB 1,2,3,6,9
Speed	X			
Flexibility	XXX			

Diving

Body Demands		Muscle Group Emphasis		Recommended Exercises
Aerobic Endurance	X	Upper Body	XX	UP 1,3,5,7
Power	XXX	Mid Body	XXX	MB 1,2,5,6,9,10
Stamina	XX	Lower Body	XX	LB 1,2,3,5,6,9
Speed	X			
Flexibility	XXX			

INDIVIDUAL COMPETITIVE SPORTS

Golf

Body Demands		Muscle Group Emphasis		Recommended Exercises
Aerobic Endurance	X	Upper Body	XX	UP 3,4,6,7,8
Power	XX	Mid Body	X	MB 5,6,9,10
Stamina	XX	Lower Body	XX	LB 2,3,6,10,12
Speed	X			
Flexibility	X			

Cycling

Body Demands		Muscle Group Emphasis		Recommended Exercises
Aerobic Endurance	XXX	Upper Body	X	UP 3,4,6,8
Power	XX	Mid Body	XX	MB 1,2,4,5
Stamina	XXX	Lower Body	XXX	LB 1,2,4,6,9,12
Speed	X			
Flexibility	X			

Skiing, Alpine

Body Demands		Muscle Group Emphasis		Recommended Exercises
Aerobic Endurance	XX	Upper Body	XX	UP 2,3,4,5,7
Power	XX	Mid Body	XX	MB 1,3,4,6,9
Stamina	XX	Lower Body	XXX	LB 1,2,4,6,7,12
Speed	XXX			
Flexibility	XX			

Weight Lifting

Body Demands		Muscle Group Emphasis		Recommended Exercises
Aerobic Endurance	X	Upper Body	XXX	UP 1,2,3,4,5,6
Power	XXX	Mid Body	XXX	MB 1,2,3,6,9
Stamina	XXX	Lower Body	XX	LB 1,2,3,4,9,12
Speed	X			
Flexibility	X			

Skiing, Cross Country

Body Demands		Muscle Group Emphasis		Recommended Exercises
Aerobic Endurance	XXX	Upper Body	XX	UP 1,3,4,5,6,7
Power	XX	Mid Body	XXX	MB 1,2,6,9,10
Stamina	XXX	Lower Body	XXX	LB 1,2,4,6,12
Speed	XX			
Flexibility	XX			

Ice Skating

Body Demands		Muscle Group Emphasis		Recommended Exercises
Aerobic Endurance	XX	Upper Body	XX	UP 3,4,5,7
Power	X	Mid Body	XX	MB 1,2,4,6,10
Stamina	XX	Lower Body	XXX	LB 1,2,4,5,6,12
Speed	XXX			
Flexibility				

COMBAT SPORTS

Boxing

Body Demands		Muscle Group Emphasis		Recommended Exercises
Aerobic Endurance	XX	Upper Body	XXX	UP 1,2,3,5,6,7
Power	XXX	Mid Body	XX	MB 1,2,3,6,9,10
Stamina	XXX	Lower Body	XXX	LB 1,2,3,9,10,12
Speed	XXX			
Flexibility	XX			

Wrestling (Freestyle and Greco-Roman)

Body Demands		Muscle Group Emphasis		Recommended Exercises
Aerobic Endurance	XX	Upper Body	XXX	UP 1,2,3,4,5,6
Power	XXX	Mid Body	XXX	MB 1,2,3,4,5,6,10
Stamina	XXX	Lower Body	XX	LB 2,3,4,6,10,12
Speed	XX			
Flexibility	XXX			

Judo

Body Demands		Muscle Group Emphasis		Recommended Exercises
Aerobic Endurance	XX	Upper Body	XXX	UP 1,2,3,4,7,8
Power	XXX	Mid Body	XX	MB 1,2,4,5,9
Stamina	XXX	Lower Body	XXX	LB 1,2,3,4,6,9,10,12
Speed	XXX			
Flexibility	XXX			

GYMNASTICS

Artistic

Body Demands		Muscle Group Emphasis		Recommended Exercises
Aerobic Endurance	X	Upper Body	XXX	UP 1,2,3,4,7,8
Power	XXX	Mid Body	XXX	MB 1,2,3,5,6,9
Stamina	XX	Lower Body	XX	LB 1,2,4,5,6,9,12
Speed	XX			
Flexibility	XXX			

Rhythmic

Body Demands		Muscle Group Emphasis		Recommended Exercises
Aerobic Endurance	XX	Upper Body	XX	UP 1,3,4,7,8
Power	XX	Mid Body	XXX	MB 1,2,6,9,10
Stamina	XX	Lower Body	XXX	LB 1,2,3,6,10,12
Speed	XX			
Flexibility	XXX			

TRACK AND FIELD EVENTS

Sprints

Aerobic Endurance	X	Upper Body	X	UP 3,5,6,7
Power	XX	Mid Body	XX	MB 1,2,4,5,9
Stamina	X	Lower Body	XXX	LB 1,2,3,4,7,10,12
Speed	XXX			
Flexibility	XX			

Hurdles

Aerobic Endurance	XX	Upper Body	X	UP 3,6,7,8
Power	XX	Mid Body	XXX	MB 1,2,4,5,6,9
Stamina	XXX	Lower Body	XXX	LB 1,2,3,4,6,9,12
Speed	XXX			
Flexibility	XXX			

Middle Distance

Aerobic Endurance	XXX	Upper Body	X	UP 3,5,6,7
Power	XXX	Mid Body	XX	MB 1,2,4,5,9
Stamina	XX	Lower Body	XXX	LB 2,3,4,7,10,12
Speed	XXX			
Flexibility	X			

Long Distance

Aerobic Endurance	XXX	Upper Body	X	UP 5,6,7,8
Power	XX	Mid Body	XXX	MB 1,2,4,5,9
Stamina	XXX	Lower Body	XXX	LB 1,2,3,6,10,12
Speed	XX			
Flexibility	X			

High Jump

Aerobic Endurance	X	Upper Body	X	UP 3,5,7,8
Power	XXX	Mid Body	XX	MB 1,2,3,4,5,9,10
Stamina	X	Lower Body	XXX	LB 1,2,3,4,6,7,12
Speed	X			
Flexibility	XX			

Long Jump

Aerobic Endurance	X	Upper Body	X	UP 1,5,6,7
Power	XXX	Mid Body	XX	MB 1,3,5,7,9
Stamina	X	Lower Body	XXX	LB 1,2,3,5,9,12
Speed	XXX			
Flexibility	XXX			

Pole Vault

Aerobic Endurance	X	Upper Body	XXX	UP 1,2,3,4,5,7,8
Power	XX	Mid Body	XXX	MB 1,2,3,5,6,9,10
Stamina	X	Lower Body	XX	LB 1,2,3,4,9,10,12
Speed	XX			
Flexibility	XX			

Shot Put

Aerobic Endurance	X	Upper Body	XXX	UP 1,2,3,4,5,6,7
Power	XXX	Mid Body	XX	MB 2,3,4,5,6,9
Stamina	XX	Lower Body	X	LB 1,2,3,6,7,9
Speed	X			
Flexibility	X			

Hammer Throw

Aerobic Endurance	X	Upper Body	XXX	UP 1,2,3,4,5,7,8
Power	XXX	Mid Body	XX	MB 1,2,3,6,9,10
Stamina	X	Lower Body	X	LB 1,2,3,6,7,9
Speed	X			
Flexibility	XX			

Discus

Aerobic Endurance	X	Upper Body	XXX	UP 1,2,3,4,5,7,8
Power	XX	Mid Body	XX	MB 1,2,3,6,9,10
Stamina	X	Lower Body	X	LB 1,2,3,6,7,9
Speed	XX			
Flexibility	XX			

Javelin

Aerobic Endurance	X	Upper Body	XXX	UP 1,2,3,4,5,7,8
Power	XX	Mid Body	XX	MB 1,2,3,6,9,10
Stamina	X	Lower Body	X	LB 1,2,3,6,7,9
Speed	XX			
Flexibility	XX			

AFTERWORD

All that any exercise can do is condition the body for the kind of training that develops the highest degrees of skill, performance, and self-confidence. There is no shortcut around good coaching and hard practice. Nor is there any shortcut around body conditioning. *As astra per aspera* ("to the stars through difficulties") the Romans used to say—and it's a long, hard road to a gold medal. But those who make it are agreed—it's worth every hour of blisters, sweat and toil, For those who can't—or don't want to—make it to the gold, the effort to attain Olympic-caliber fitness is an investment that pays dividends for the rest of your life.